CHANGE YOUR GRIP ON LIFE THROUGH TENNIS!

A Player's Physical, Mental, Technical, & Nutritional Guide for Improving Your Game

Carmen Micsa

Wistful Press

CARMICHAEL, CA

Copyright © 2016 by **Carmen Micsa**

All rights reserved. No part of this publication may be reproduced, distributed or transmitted in any form or by any means, without prior written permission.

**Carmen Micsa/Wistful Press
6100 Fair Oaks Blvd., Suite A3
Carmichael, Ca 95608
www.carmenmicsabooks.com**

Book Layout © 2014 BookDesignTemplates.com

Change Your Grip on Life Through Tennis/Carmen Micsa. - 1st ed.
ISBN 978-0-9983097-1-2 (eBook)
ISBN 978-0-9983097-5 (paperback)

Dedication

This book is dedicated to my dear father Danut Gramatic, who bought me a wooden racket when I was 12 in Lugoj, Romania. Even though the court in front of our apartment was without a net, we still played tennis. Playing tennis and soccer with my father will always be one of my most treasured memories about him. I also dedicate this book to my mother who supports my passion for sports and always believes in me.

It is also dedicated to my wonderful husband Catalin Micsa, who is my mixed doubles partner and who always beats me in singles. Through his athleticism and focus, he helps me become a better competitor, as he always makes me hit one more shot before winning or losing the point.

Finally, I dedicate this book to our sweet children, Alex and Sophia, who love to exercise and enjoy basketball and gymnastics. Our children are my reason to exercise, stay healthy, and strive for excellence. They support my love of tennis and are proud of their mother.

Acknowledgements

Special thanks to all my tennis coaches who have helped me become a better player and human being. A million thanks to Betsy Kessing, my very first coach, Yemi Tallman, Milun Doskovic, Amine Khalid, Reed Stout, Jason Johnson, Glen Davis, Martin Kosan, and everyone who gave me tips on improving my technique and taking my tennis game to the next level.

A million thanks to my outstanding editor Theresa Warren, who has been the most helpful, positive, and brilliant editor I could have asked for. I am extremely grateful for the day we met on the tennis court and had a great match. Not only do we have tennis in common, but we also share the love of English and writing.

Many thanks to my outstanding cover designer, Kellie W Patterson, who put a lot of hard work and passion to make my book look great.

And last, but not least, a heartfelt thank you to my amazing friend Jenni Wiltz, an award-winning author, who has helped and guided me through the entire book publishing process. You can find her books at http://JenniWiltz.com.

Introduction

"Nothing great was ever achieved without enthusiasm."

Ralph Waldo Emerson

When I first started playing tennis, I never stretched, did weight lifting, or ran/cross trained. After more than twenty years of playing tennis and a lot of personal research, I decided to share my insights, my transformation, and my tips with other players so they could have access to my concise tennis compendium. It was only after fifteen years that I started to take my tennis game more seriously and appreciated the physical, mental, and spiritual side of tennis. In order to take my tennis game to the next level, I decided to join the American River College team and played for them in the 2014 season. During that season, I learned to properly warm-up, stretch, run, and lift light weights. This gave me a new perspective on tennis, which I wanted to share with other players.

Additionally, I thought that being an amateur league and tournament tennis player and not a high-ranked professional, would make my book more relatable to other dedicated recreational players' journeys. The purpose is to provide useable knowledge on topics such as: cross-training, nutrition, and tennis equipment that has been experienced by other amateur players. Player-to-player advice is competing at tennis for fun, as well as competitively in USTA's (United States Tennis Association) leagues and tournaments.

Tennis has changed my perspective on life and has helped me become more positive, confident, focused, and happier. It has also transformed me physically, emotionally, spiritually, and mentally, which is why I keep researching and learning new aspects of the game. It was my goal to rise above mediocrity in tennis and life and try to achieve my highest potential.

This book represents my own personal tennis journey. I started as a self-rated 3.5 player in 1999. My husband Catalin and I played tennis for fun beginning in 1995 when we came to this wonderful country and marveled at the free tennis courts, which is uncommon in Europe. After many trials and tribulations, the USTA moved me up to the 4.5 level in 2015. This was also the year that I played my best tennis and finished number 2 in Northern California in
women's 4.0 singles and number three in mixed doubles that I played with my husband.

My success came from applying the lessons learned from my American River College coach Reed Stout and many other coaches I have taken lessons from throughout the years. I am humbled by this long journey, and even though I am not an authority on tennis, nutrition, exercise, I have identified these ten assets that qualify me to write about my tennis and life success during my journey.

1. A B.A. and M.A in English (creative writing).

2. A published author.

3. Completion of over 100 USTA tournaments.

4. I have played tennis for 20+ years and still learning something new about this beautiful game.

5. A black belt in Taekwondo.

6. I breathe, eat, and sleep tennis.

7. A strong grasp of the mental aspect of the game, as well as its application to our lives.

8. I am a marathon and ultra marathon runner and believe in fitness and cross training.

9. Confidence that tennis players of all levels can find great strategies to become better tennis players and human beings.

10. I am a regular tennis player just like you who wants to share lessons learned to make your tennis experience smoother, more fun, and more rewarding.

Therefore, this book is perfect for the novice, intermediate, and advanced amateur tennis players, as well as junior players, other athletes, or anyone who enjoys fitness and exercise because of the cross training, fitness, and nutrition chapters. It can also provide a great insight to parents who want their children to enjoy playing tennis for fun or to obtain scholarships through tennis achievement.

I hope you will enjoy reading this book, and that you, too, will achieve a higher ranking, as well as make good use of the invaluable life lessons *that* tennis teaches us.

Play and win with **LOVE**! Stay **humbled and grounded**: my favorite mantra that I use during matches. And last, but not least, remember: "tennis is life," so live life to the fullest! Carpe Diem!

Contents

Copyright 2

Dedication 3

Acknowledgements 5

Introduction 7

Chapter One: Change 13

Chapter Two: Learning and Topspin 19

Chapter Three: Early Preparation and Slice 23

Chapter Four: Tennis Drills 27

Chapter Five: Drills and Exercises for a Stronger, Faster You 37

Chapter Six: Cross Training and Conditioning 49

Chapter Seven: Breathing, Balance, and Staying Grounded 59

Chapter Eight: Speed and Split Steps 69

Chapter Nine: The Zen of Tennis 73

Chapter Ten: Mental Focus and Concentration 81

Chapter Eleven: Play Loose and Relaxed - Serve It Up! 87

Chapter Twelve: Embrace Change by Playing Singles and Doubles 93

Chapter Thirteen: Expand Your Tennis Toolbox with a Variety of Shots and Strokes 101

Chapter Fourteen: Rackets and Strings 105

Chapter Fifteen: Got Grips? Tennis and Life Grips 113

Chapter Sixteen: Eating a Balanced Diet - Proper Nutrition 119

Chapter Seventeen: Carmen's Fresh, Easy, and Healthy Menus and Recipes 129

Chapter Eighteen: Tips and Lessons to Take Your Tennis Game to the Next Level 137

Chapter Nineteen: The College Experience: a Faster, Fun, and Rewarding Way to Move up the Tennis Ladder 147

Chapter Twenty: The PR of Tennis 153

Chapter Twenty-One: Carmen's 100 Life Lessons 159

Tennis Resources 165

Works Cited 173

About the Author 175

CHAPTER ONE

Change

"I like to be in the creative spirit all the time. Everybody is moving – the people, our planet – you either keep up with it or you just stay where you are… But if you stay wherever you are, you actually regress."

Novak Djokovic

John C. Maxwell's quote "change is inevitable, growth is optional" epitomizes the key to getting better at everything we do, whether it is becoming better parents, professionals, friends, writers, athletes, or simply better tennis players. Albert Einstein also made a valuable point with his statement: "doing the same thing over and over again and expecting different results is the definition of insanity." This premise lays the groundwork for my objective to try and change your grip on life by changing your approach to a winning tennis game.

Let's embark on a journey of transformation together by emerging out of our comfortable cocoons and disrupting complacency! If you don't like the word change, use "tweak", "adjustment," or anything else that will help you improve as a person and tennis player. Do whatever it takes to get motivated. Refuse to be one of many recreational players who takes a ton of lessons from tennis pros, and yet, resists change.

How can your game improve if you are not ready to change your grip? Grip is imperative to learning slice or topspin strokes. Learning how to change your grip will assure adding new shots that will result in more flexibility and variety in your game.

When I played a few 4.5 tournaments in 2013, I took lessons from various tennis pros who each added a new dimension to my game. They worked with me to develop a topspin forehand, make my backhand stronger, and change my serve. After having learned three forehands, slice, topspin, and reverse topspin, or what many call "Nadal's forehand" and two backhands, I became a more versatile player and took my game to the next level. Although my USTA rating was only 4.0, I finished number two in Northern California in the 4.5 singles. I lost the Grand Prix final to a good 4.5 player, but played well and welcomed the tougher competition.

The year of 2014 was my biggest learning curve year. I played for American River College team and had a blast learning new strokes and strategies about the game. The year 2015 proved to be my best year in tennis, as I finally got moved up to 4.5, a higher level in USTA (United States Tennis Association). All my tennis lessons had finally synced and cumulated in me. This new understanding of the game helped me be undefeated in tournaments and leagues for the first half of the year in Northern California. I finished number two in Northern California tennis tournaments (NCTA). I also played the Grand Prix in women singles, women doubles 4.5, and mixed doubles with my husband.

Some of the primary improvements I made were these:

1. **Serving** (not hopping like a bunny anymore when serving).

2. **Hitting my slice with a Continental grip** instead of Eastern.

3. **Stronger two-handed topspin backhand.**

4. **Adding topspin** to my game for versatility and variety.

5. **Changing my racket to Babolat Pure Drive** and changing my strings to add more spin.

Even with the best instruction, great results are always dependent on the players' dedication to practicing new strokes. Pro Amine Khaldi from Gold River Racket Club taught me for almost a year. He diligently worked with me to develop a topspin forehand and backhand that would add to my arsenal of tennis strokes. He used various contraptions and equipment to teach me the appropriate arm and leg positions for proper execution of a topspin stroke. Yet, my reluctance to use the strokes in competition and practice my newly learned topspin strokes resulted in less application of topspin in my game.

I also remember the lesson I took from Glenn Davis, a wonderful tennis pro from Natomas Racket Club. He taught me the acceleration on the forehand by having me hit a towel as hard and fast as I could. He also had me use the towel to pretend that I was hitting the ball to create a loose feeling in my arm and body. The relaxed feeling of hitting the ball can only come from constant repetition and not worrying about winning the point. The more we practice what we learn, the easier it is to relax and trust those shots.

Striving to win in competition was inhibiting my ability to practice new strategies and strokes pros had worked hard to help me learn. I decided I needed a different tennis environment that would provide more opportunities to expand my game. A good friend of mine, Tamra, invited me to join the American River College team. Taking a couple of classes at the college qualified me to join the team. Even though Tamra encouraged me to join, it was a conversation with another tournament friend, Sara, who assured me it could be a good move for my tennis game. Her topspin ground strokes were so impressive. I had to comment.

"You have such amazing topspin and ground strokes," I told Sara.

"That's because my husband and I used to play for a college team. We learned so much, as we were more mature than the other kids on the team and the coach really liked us," she recalled smiling at the pleasant experience that trickled over the net of life.

"Wow! You can do that?" I remember asking her. "Be on the college team?" Sara asked. "Of course! Almost anybody can, especially on the women's teams."

A big light bulb went off in my brain! If I didn't seize this opportunity, I could choose to be ripe and rotten, as Jason Johnson, another of my amazing tennis coaches, told me, or I could stay green and ripe. On the other hand, being a mother, made me seriously consider this game plan. Playing tennis for a college team to get better at a sport I should enjoy just for the exercise and social aspect seemed self-indulging. This would definitely take time away from my family. I was a good 4.0 player, but I aspired to become 4.5 USTA rated player, and higher. Despite the time commitment, my husband agreed and truly encouraged me to embark on this journey. I am so glad I did not listen to the doubting and guilty voices in my head.

Key points

1. Got grip? **Check your grip** and see if it needs tweaking.

2. **Embrace change**.

3. **Find two or three different coaches**. Get different opinions and suggestions to become a better player.

4. **Find a coach who understands your game**, is more demanding, and asks you to make changes rather than offering empty praise.

5. **Take detailed notes** after each lesson.

6. **Have a tennis notebook** in which you jot down strategies, technique, shot selections, etc. Take notes on the players you played against. It will help you strategize the next time you play against them, especially if you lost.

7. **Apply your lessons** through easy drills.

8. **Play against various level players**. It will help you work on your game and see the improvement faster.

9. **Play league matches and tournaments**. Practice against different opponents and challenge yourself.

10. **Repeat, repeat, and repeat** to gain confidence and proficiency in your shots.

CHAPTER TWO

Learning and Topspin

"Tennis begins with love."

Author Unknown

In August 2013, I went back to school to a twice-a-week tennis class that would prepare me for being on the college team during the 2014 season. I immediately liked our coach Reed Stout, and seeing my friend Tamra's smiling face there made me feel more at home amidst all the 20-year-olds who would soon find out from me that I was there just for the pure joy of tennis. I already had a Master's degree in English (Creative Writing). The classes were just for me to continue to grow and learn, and, most importantly, to be eligible to play on the team.

Coach Reed Stout liked my slices, but immediately sprang into action to teach me an effective topspin, which I knew I had to learn and was ready. He emphasized that turning my body fast was key. He stressed not to lunge or lean while striking the ball. Although I was fast at running balls down, coach Reed taught me to run behind the ball, then move forward to increase momentum and power. This resulted in hitting a bigger and better shot. Yet, my continued desire to learn how to hit a good topspin meant comprehending and breaking down the topspin moves.

Having already had instruction from Pro Khaldi on the execution of topspin strokes, the concept seemed clear. The term "windshield wiper" used to describe the topspin stroke was quite familiar to me. Yet, my idea of good topspin changed once I grasped that the power and effectiveness of a solid topspin depended on the legs and rotation of the body. I took notes and paid attention to my posture, footwork, early preparation, and staying grounded. The fundamentals to good topspin are bending the knees, staying low, and straightening up the body as we hit through the shot without jumping. The legs and hips create the power to hit solid topspin. I also learned to really place the ball. When I took the ball a little bit in front, I could easily execute a crosscourt topspin shot. When I waited for the ball to come closer to my body, I could hit a down the line shot.

One of the things we need to learn as tennis players is to use our legs a lot more than our arms. This advice that Coach Reed gave me was paramount to becoming a better player and hitting better topspin. I also learned that guiding or pushing the balls in, instead of relying on a wider stance and good leg power, weakened my game. It may sound confusing, and you're probably thinking: "Hey! I thought I was playing tennis, not soccer." However, power in tennis comes from the ground.

Try to think you're a powerful twister. As you rotate your hips into the ball, you will gain more power in your stroke. Using my legs and hips felt as strange as climbing stairs on my hands. Although I have a black belt in Taekwondo and learned to smash through boards with good hip rotation, tennis seemed to be about strong arms that could help me power the ball to the other side of the net. I have learned to let go of this misconceived idea. Being a self-taught tennis player, I knew that I needed a new grip, stroke, and a new perspective. The mind needed to control my jumpy and explosive body that wanted to levitate when hitting shots, which was the wrong way to create power.

I thus understood that in order to strike the ball well, I had to plant my feet and rotate my hips through the shot, while fully extending my arm. Hitting the ball in balance had to match my inner harmony, while there was no rush other than getting to the ball and planting my feet. Gripping life in its stillness. Finding the peace and calmness of playing with a Zen-like mind.

Key points about topspin:

1. Get your body in position. **Early preparation**.

2. **Turn your upper body**, shoulder, your entire unit.

3. **Stay grounded,** as if your legs are one with the surface whether it's hard-court, clay, or grass.

4. **Loosen the grip on your racket.** Don't tighten the arm while hitting, as you're only stopping the flow. There is a reason everything we learn teaches us to go with the flow, or not swim against the current.

5. **Wait for the ball** to get in your striking zone (hip level).

6. **Take the arm back and go through your shot.** Hitting is the last thing that needs to happen, although our eager natures tell us to hit, hit, and hit some more.

Key points about learning:

1. Approach everything with an **open mind**.

2. **Be curious**.

3. **Be excited to learn something new**.

4. **Dismiss fear** and doubts and plow through.

5. **Practice what you learn** and implement it.

6. **Don't make excuses about your age!** It is never too late to learn something new.

7. Learning something new is not always easy, but **do not give up!**

8. **Set higher goals for yourself**, instead of being content with less.

9. Make it a goal **to learn something new every day**.

10. **Enjoy the journey**, go with the flow, and choose the path of learning.

CHAPTER THREE

Early Preparation and Slice

"Proper preparation prevents poor performance."

Charlie Batch

To adapt Charlie Batch's quote to tennis, I would say: "early preparation prevents poor performance."

I have decided to devote a special chapter on preparation and slice for two reasons: preparation is the most difficult aspect of the game for me to apply (I am almost always late turning my body and preparing to hit the ball) and slice is my signature shot, my strength, and my uniqueness that will make players remember me after playing a match.

The early preparation in tennis is one of the most quintessential components that will help you become successful on and off the court. Whether you play tennis for fun or competition, once you have understood and applied the concept of early preparation, which simply means to react as soon as the ball leaves your opponent's strings and to meet the ball with balance and equilibrium, you are setting yourself up for success in tennis and life. Any time you are prepared and do not allow your opponent to make you feel rushed, you position yourself to be in control, to hit the right shot, and to be mindful.

Due to the fact that when I started playing tennis, I hit most of the shots with an open stance and reacted to the ball at the last minute, changing my bad habit of late or no preparation felt insurmountable. My very first coach Betsy Kessing suggested I changed my grip from Eastern to Continental, which gave me more depth and consistency. Another coach, Glen Davis, who liked my slices when I did clinics and private lessons with him, noticed something different and said to me:

"The reason you miss some of your sliced forehands is because you wait till the last moment to hit the ball and you are not ready. You need to act like a baseball player."

"I don't know anything about baseball, coach," I replied.

"Well, it's simple. Do you see the catcher catch the ball at the last minute, or do you see him with the hand in front, getting ready to track and catch the ball?"

"Oh, I get it," I said while pretending to grasp the foreign concept of baseball. "I need to be in position sooner and not wait till the last minute to hit the ball, right, coach?"

"Precisely," he replied, waving his arms up and down, as if to put a halt on the late preparation and reaction from me on the court.

Coach Davis got to work. In just one lesson, my preparation and execution of a more effective and deeper slice improved and helped me become a more consistent player. From then on, my slices had become meaner and meaner, as most players I played against told me. Not only did I have a lot of backspin on the ball, but my slices stayed very low, making it hard for my opponents to hit good topspin, as they had to really bend down to get to the ball.

As my coaches pointed out how my body position and footwork affected my slice, I understood more about my game, so I set out to refine my slices by mixing up the spinning slices with my driving ones.

Spinning Slices:

To hit a spinning slice, I would just carve the ball more, which meant going underneath the ball and moving my right hand in a scooping motion, as if painting a U out of thin air. These type of slices are particularly effective when executing a drop shot, or hitting a short angle slice, as the ball spins away from your opponent and the bounce just dies down.

Driving Slices:

Driving slices are my signature shots, especially the ones I hit down the line from my deuce side to my opponent's ad side. To hit a good driving slice that goes deep into the court, I turn my body early (when I don't forget or I am not too lazy), hit the ball sideways, and drive through the ball.

More key points to developing an effective slice:

1. **Continental grip** is the most effective and common way to hit a great slice.

2. **Be prepared to change grips** when hitting a slice.

3. **Early preparation is key**, so turn your body and be ready.

4. When hitting a slice, **your body is turned sideways.**

5. As you hit a slice, **your body needs to move forward.**

6. **Do not lunge for the ball**, or you will hit the ball into the net!

7. You see pros hit slices mainly when they are stretched and on defense, but **being in good position will help you hit a deeper and more offensive slice.**

8. To hit an effective slice, **you need to be close to the ball and balanced.**

9. You hear coaches repeat **"step into the ball"** for most shots; this is especially helpful when returning topspin by hitting a slice, as moving your body forward will generate more power, depth, and spin on the ball.

10. As you finish hitting your slice, **do not open your stance**. Stay sideways and follow your shot.

CHAPTER FOUR

Tennis Drills

"The depressing thing about tennis is that no matter how good I get, I'll never be as good as a wall."

Mitch Hedberg

We have all heard a million times the word practice, or the expression "practice makes it better." In tennis, just like in other sports, drills are basic to training and improving specific techniques in the sport. The benefits of using drills to improve my game have not only been far-reaching, but provided an opportunity for me to develop personalized drills customized to my needs. This chapter is dedicated to "drills" I have learned from coaches and others that I have created, or have mixed from the drills I learned, especially from my American River College coach, Reed Stout. I'd like to begin with my drills which are titled, "Carmen's Drills."

CARMEN'S DRILLS:

The smacking power of tennis is both overestimated and underestimated amongst tennis players of all levels. When I was 12 years old and started playing tennis with my father, I was merely interested in pushing the ball back across the net with my wooden racket. I was happy to just strike the ball, not thinking about power. When we overestimate the driving power we can produce with modern rackets, we forget about taking the pace off the ball by choosing to use slice, drop shot, high topspin, or moon balls, and so on. Thus, the following drills are designed to help you rethink your tennis game, as well as help you become a smarter, more strategic, more purposeful and well-rounded player.

1.   Short court drill.

Purpose: To improve control on the ball, as well as add finesse to your game.

Hit short balls with various spins topspin and slice, or underhand inside the service box down the line. Focus on hitting at least 10 balls in a row by using various spins and angles. Work on touch and control. The objective is to practice control of low power shots.

2.   Short court, angles drill.

Purpose: Develop more of a geometric thinking on the court and improve your angle shots.

This is the same drill as the one above. However, this time go cross court and focus even more on angles. Goal is to hit 10 balls in a row and get to 20 once you are very consistent, but you can start with four shots if you are still new to the game.

3. Carmen's two-shot spin drill.

Purpose: Shot selection and variation, as well as to give your opponent a different spin on the ball and force errors.

Practice hitting the ball with various spins. Hit a topspin followed by a slice down the middle of the court. As you warm-up both shots, hit your two shots cross court, and end the drill by hitting one topspin and one slice down the line. Many players are very good at handling the same type of ball, but have trouble adjusting their footwork when given a different shot. Shot variation will take your game to the next level faster.

4. The wall drill.

Purpose: Consistency and mental toughness.

For beginners and advanced players, make the wall your friend. When I was 12, my father and I started to play tennis, but I also wanted to practice on my own, so I used the side of our apartment complex as my wall. I remember how a few times I hit the ball all the way to our neighbors' balconies and even knocked down a potted plant one time. I ran away afraid to face my angry neighbors, yet promising the wall I would come back.

My wall drill is very simple: you need to start with one shot and then hit as many shots consistently in a row as possible. I always felt victorious if I could get to 20 shots in a row. Hitting one more ball, assures one more shot, which could make the difference in winning or losing the point against tough opponents. It also strengthens mental toughness and focus.

5. Serving drill.

Purpose: Flexibility in use of different serves.

Hit four different serves on each side. Hit flat, topspin, slice, and kick serves. Serve variation is key in winning tough matches against opponents with good returns (See the chapter on serving to learn all four type of serves).

6. Carmen's serve and volley drill.

Purpose: Learning to track the ball and react after serving.

a. If you really want to put your opponents on the defensive, learn to serve and volley. Find a partner who wants to work on the same technique. Follow the same rules of ping-pong where each player serves five times. In this drill, you begin by serving and volleying at least two times. If you don't come to the net, you automatically lose the game.

b. The second part of this drill is to serve and volley four times out of five regardless of the outcome. In this second part of the drill, really focus on serving and try mixing up different serves. The ideal way to set yourself up for a winning shot is to serve to the "T" (backhand on players who are right-handed), serve to the body, or serve wide. Mixing kick serves with slices and topspins is very important to be successful at serve and volley.

7. Carmen's never miss drill.

Purpose: Consistency, focus, and turning into a "human wall" that will frustrate opponents.

To practice this drill, find another consistent player and work on spins rather than power to keep the ball in the court for as long as possible. Ideally, you can hit at least 30 balls in a row, but for the sake of this drill, both you and your partner count how many shots you can hit and always raise the bar to go for longer rallies in case you will need them in a match. Endurance is our friend in tennis. We can easily tire out our opponents by being consistent and working the point. Perseverance is also an ally as ball after ball, we keep hitting with depth and placement to exhaust our opponents both mentally and physically. This is one of Novak Djokovic's best strategies in tough matches. He plays solid tennis and draws unforced errors from his opponents, even when he is not hitting the ball as hard as he could, although he hits it deep.

8. The slice drill.

Purpose: Changing the pace, keeping the ball low so that your opponent has a hard time attacking it.

In this drill, you only hit slice forehands and backhands starting short and then moving to the baseline. To hit effective slices, turn your body, step into the ball, and drive the ball with a slice by going from high to low, the opposite motion of topspin.

Even though today's tennis relies heavily on the topspin stroke, adding slice to your game will give you an advantage over most tennis players. Slice adds variety to your game and forces your opponents out of their comfort zone. Alternating your shots will force your opponent to change grip and footwork. Preparation is totally different when hitting a topspin shot vs. a slice shot. I won at least five matches 6-0, 6-0 when playing for my college team, because the players I played against had no idea how to handle my slice, even though they had very good topspin. Find a coach who still sees value in slice and can teach you how to do it correctly. The best way to add slice into your game is by changing your grip to continental (see the chapter on slice for details on executing the shot).

9. The drop shot - lob drill.

Purpose: This drill helps you practice the control of utilizing a drop shot while preparing for a lob over your opponent.

Focus on hitting a drop shot to bring your opponent in. Then, imagine your opponent between the service line and net and execute a lob. This drill will help you take control of points where you feel it is hard to compete against a good baseline player.

10. The one - two punch drill.

Purpose: To practice winning the point in two shots.

You will serve wide, after which you will hit the ball down the line for a winner. This drill is particularly effective, as most players will return a wide serve cross court. They are pulled off the court wide leaving the open court available for a down-the-line shot, which is most used in singles.

Other drills learned from American River College coach Reed and other pros:

1. **Hit cross court to cross court** with heavy spin.

2. **Hit cross court using only slices** on both deuce and ad sides.

3. **Figure 8s** - where one player hits cross court and the other player hits down the line. They switch roles after five minutes.

4. **Practice hitting deep balls** by playing a groundstroke game, where if you hit the ball in the service box, you lose the point.

5. **The mixed groundstroke drill** - Play a groundstroke game where one person feeds the ball.

6. **A defensive high moon ball to the other player's backhand**. Work the point aggressively, but with consistency. The other player should not take a defensive approach and back up way behind the baseline. Instead, she should commit to taking the ball early and make a good, deep return cross court. Play to 11, using a tie break format. The goal is to dictate the points, make the match physical, while playing solid and consistent tennis that will force the opponent to return a short ball for you to put away.

7. **The rapid fire drill** - Practice hitting as many forehands as possible in a speedy manner that requires early preparation, turning your shoulders and body, bearing weight on the right leg for right-handed players, and ripping the ball.

8. **Hitting down the line drill** - Working on balance and long arm extension. Alleys are good.

9. **The overhead drill** - Practice four overheads from the service line and four from the baseline. Stand up straight with shoulders turned and don't drop your shoulders.

10. **The "Blood and Guts drill"** - Play a game to help your doubles game, where everybody is at the service line and the players move together closer and closer to the net. No lobs allowed and a clear winner down the middle gives you two points. Play up to 15 or 21.

11. **The shot variation drill** - One player hits with heavy topspin and the other player hits high looping topspin, or moon balls.

12. **The deep shot drill**, where both players have to hit deep shots. The players who hits the ball short by the service line, loses the point.

13. **The net drill**, where the player who wins the point from the net with a volley or overhead, earns two points.

14. **The slice and topspin drill** - One player hits slices only and the other player hits topspins.

15. **The slice and moon ball drill** - One player hits slices and the other player hits moon balls in order to develop a variety of shots.

16. **The "dink-em" drill** - This drill works for both singles and doubles. For singles, use half the court no alleys. For doubles use half the court and the alleys. Everybody starts at the net

and dinks the ball over. The ball will need to bounce once, after which the other team plays the ball. Angles and soft touches are key in this drill.

17. **Volley drills**: one player starts back feeding the ball, while the other one moves in and keeps making volleys. This is played on half a court, including the alley, but it goes cross court to cross court starting by the service line on the deuce side, then ad side to ad side. Play up to 11.

18. Another drill is **feeding the ball to the net player** who has to take all balls out of the air, or the point is lost.

19. **In this volley drill, one player catches the ball first on her racket, and then she makes the volley**. This is a great drill to develop finesse and soft touch volleys. Someone needs to feed you balls, as you keep doing this for 10 to 15 times till you "feel" the volley.

20. One player feeds **volleys from the middle of the court** and the other player who starts crosscourt, hits volleys in the air. While hitting the next volley, the player keeps crossing and moving to the other side of the court. You start on the deuce side and you end up on the ad side by the service line, or vice-a-versa. This is perfect for developing confidence in one's poaching abilities.

Key points:

1. **Focus on specific shots**, such as forehand or backhand.

2. **Learn various shots**, such as topspins and slices.

3. **Practice volleys and overheads**, as well as play singles and doubles to make you a more versatile player.

4. **Practice being consistent** by making Carmen's Never Miss Drill part of your routine.

5. **Make the wall your best tennis friend**. It will still defeat you, but you will become a wall in matches and beat a lot of your frustrated opponents.

6. **Improve your serve** by learning and practicing flat serves, topspins, kick serves, and slices.

Always persevere!

CHAPTER FIVE

Drills and Exercises for a Stronger, Faster You

"While other sports can provide excellent health benefits and some can promote mental and emotional growth, none can compete with tennis in delivering overall physical, mental, and emotional gains."

Jack Groppel, former chairman of the USTA's National Sport Science Committee

Having success on the tennis court includes more than a variety of shots and consistency in your game. Fitness is ultimately important to winning. Without it, the shots will suffer and consistency is jeopardized. Once you have learned a variety of tennis shots and feel that you are becoming a good tennis player, you need to go to the next level of fitness in your game. I have included some agility and footwork drills that you can immediately incorporate in your routine. There is also a wide selection of exercises, so please don't feel overwhelmed and think that you need to quit your job and spend all your time on training. All these drills are designed to help you perform better and stay injury free. The variety will give you the option of choosing and creating your own routine.

Agility and footwork drills:

1. **Side-hop exercise** – Place a small gym bag or any other stable object on a firm surface. Stand directly to the side of it. Keeping your feet together, side-hop like a bunny over the object back and forth, for one minute.

2. **Split-step exercise** - One person throws the ball to the other who has to catch the ball in the air or with one bounce only. Split-step between running from one side to another. Split-step means a quick stop before making the next move. This allows you to move left or right just like on the tennis court when making volleys. Do 24 of these ball throw/catch exercises and mix them up with short, wide, and middle balls just like on the tennis court. Try to get in three sets of these and in between, do lunges.

3. **Foot speed drills using the stairs** - Step left foot onto stair. Immediately step right foot onto step while simultaneously returning left foot to start. Move lightning fast.

4. **Running** - Intense running for a quarter mile.

Core exercises and drills:

Does your lower back hurt you after playing a long and tough match? Mine used to hurt a lot until I started to practice martial arts at Carmichael Family Taekwondo. While training there for my black belt, I learned how to do proper push-ups, sit-ups, and lunges, which strengthened my core and made my lower back pain disappear. Here's a suggested routine:

1. Start your morning with **20 pushups and 20 sit-ups**, even if you have no time to add any other exercises that day.

2. Do **mountain climbers** by being in push-up position and bringing knees to your chest, one at a time.

3. **Twisters** - Start lying face-up on the floor, holding your legs in the air perpendicular to the floor, your legs straight, and your arms extended outward like wings resting on the floor. Keeping your shoulders and arms anchored to the floor and your legs together, swing your legs over to your left side. Touch your left foot to the floor to mark a complete repetition. Keeping your shoulders and arms anchored to the floor and your legs together, bring your legs 180 degrees over to your right side. Touch your right foot to the floor to mark another repetition. Return your legs to the starting position.

4. **Plank** for 30 seconds to two minutes, one of the best core strengthening exercises. Start in a facedown position, propped up on your elbows, with your elbows aligned directly beneath your shoulders and your forearms resting on the floor. Your knees should be fully extended and your toes on the floor. Squeeze your gluts, draw your belly button in toward your spine and raise your hips approximately one foot above the floor. Your body should be rigid and elevated

from heels to shoulders. Hold the position as long as you can. Lower hips to the ground when you need to rest.

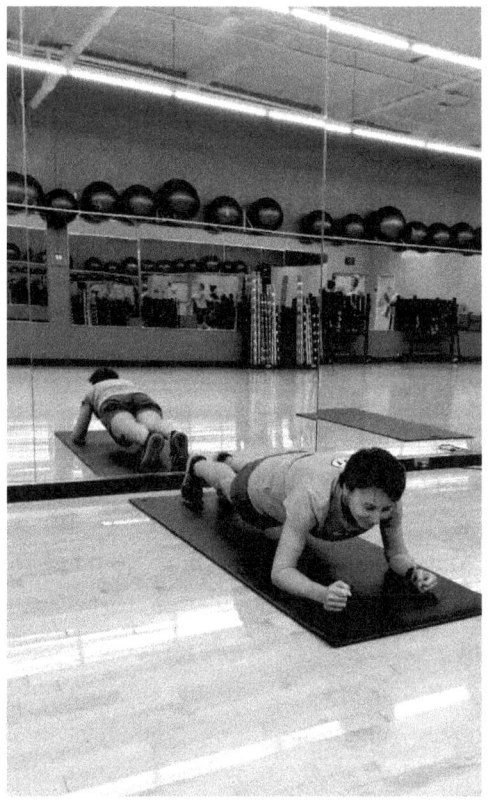

5. Do one minute of **burpees**. The correct way to do burpees is to stand with your feet shoulder-width apart. Squat all the way down, placing your hands on the floor. Supporting your weight on your hands, kick your feet back into a plank position and do a pushup. Pull your legs back into a squat, and then jump straight up in the air. Burpees are considered the best exercises for tennis players, as they help with explosiveness on the court.

6. Do 20 seconds to 40 seconds of **squats**. The correct way to do them is to have your feet hip-width apart, after which you stick your glutes out towards your imaginary chair.

7. **Lunges**, such as basic ones, when you make a big step far back with the right leg stretched out and sink your body low putting weight on your leg. The correct way of doing lunges is to keep your torso erect without letting your back knee touch the ground. Repeat 10-20 repetitions and then switch legs. For more intensity, carry weights in your hands or on your shoulders.

8. **Glute bridges** are quite important, since the most explosives moves come from your hips, and often times tennis players do not strengthen them. You start by lying down on the floor. You bend your legs and bring your feet close to your glutes. Pull your body up in a bridge and then lower. Repeat 10 times.

Besides the above-mentioned exercises, according to the running expert, Christine Luff, these exercises should be excellent core and strengthening routines in the life of any athlete who wants to avoid injuries.

Below please find some suggested routines for athletes. As always, you need to carefully begin these exercises to see what your body can endure. Everyone is different and some muscle groups may be better developed than others. You may have to build up to regular use of these routines.

Description of the routines below and how to do them correctly:

1. **Wall sit** is great in building a strong core and balance. To do this, simply pretend you are sitting in an imaginary chair with your back against the wall. Keep your back straight and feet apart and in a good balance to create this chair pose. Breathe in and out and tighten your core muscles.

2. **Bicycle crunches** are great for the abdominal and the oblique muscles. To do them correctly, you will need to lie flat on the floor with your lower back pressed to the ground (pull your navel in to also target your deep abs). Put your hands behind your head, then bring your knees in towards your chest and lift your shoulder blades off the ground, but be sure not to pull on your neck. Straighten your right leg out to about a 45-degree angle to the ground while turning your upper body to the left, bringing your right elbow towards the left knee. Make sure your rib cage is moving and not just your elbows. Don't forget to switch sides and do the same motion on the other side to complete one rep.

3. **Reverse Crunches** target the lower abdominal muscles. Lie down on your back and put your arms behind your head. With knees off the ground bring them towards your forehead without moving the head or shoulders. It is just a slight movement that will engage the lower abdominal muscles.

4. **Bird Dog** is another excellent exercise to tighten your abdominal muscles. Start from all four position. Slowly extend your left leg behind you while reaching your right

arm forward. Keep your hips and shoulders square and make sure your lower back doesn't arch. Hold for five seconds. Slowly return to the starting position and do the move on the opposite side.

5. **Superman exercises** are great to strengthen the abs and lower back. First, lie down on a mat or flat surface with arms outstretched, as if flying. Keep your hands and arms straight throughout the exercise. Raise your hand and legs 4-5 inches off the ground for 5 seconds. Return to starting position.

BEGINNER:

Lower body focus:

- 15 squats
- 15 lunges (on each side)
- Wall sit (hold 30 seconds, repeat 3 times)
- 3 x 10 heel raises (10 in each position – feet parallel, toes pointing out, toes pointing in)
- 10 toe raises

Core work:

- Front plank (hold 30 seconds)
- Side plank (both sides, hold 30 seconds)
- Bicycle crunch (one minute)
- 12 Bird dog (hold 5 seconds)
- Reverse crunch (30 seconds)
- 20 push-ups

Once the above routine becomes too easy, you can progress to the intermediate, and then advanced routines:

INTERMEDIATE:

The first number stands for the set. So 2 x 15 squats means two sets of 15 squats. Take a 30-second break between sets to shake out your muscles and/or get a drink of water.

Lower body focus:

- 2 x 15 squats
- 2 x 15 lunges (on each side)
- Wall sit hold 40 seconds, repeat 3 times)
- 3 x 10 heel raises (10 in each position – feet parallel, toes pointing out, toes pointing in)
- 15 toe raises

Core work:

- Front plank (hold 45 seconds)
- Side plank (both sides, hold 45 seconds)
- Bicycle crunch (90 seconds)
- 12 Bird dog (hold 10 seconds)
- Reverse crunch (one minute)
- 40 push-ups
- Superman (hold 3 seconds x 5)

ADVANCED:

The first number stands for the set. 3 x 15 squats means three sets of 15 squats. Take a 30-second break between sets to shake out your muscles and/or get a drink of water.

Lower body focus:

- 3 x 15 squats
- 3 x 10 lunges (on each side)
- Wall sit (hold 45 seconds, repeat 3 times)
- 3 x 10 heel raises (10 in each position – feet parallel, toes pointing out, toes pointing in)
- 2 x 10 toe raises

Core work:

- Front planks (hold 60-90 seconds)
- Side plank (both sides, hold 60-90 seconds)
- Bicycle crunch (2 minutes)
- 12 Bird dog (hold 15 seconds)
- Reverse crunch (90 seconds)
- 50 push-ups
- Superman (hold 5 seconds x 10)

Carmen's Top Five daily exercises for a stronger, faster YOU:

1. Push-ups – 20 every morning before I start my day.

2. Lunges – 20.

3. Squats – 20 or more. I do them throughout the day while cooking, standing, taking a break from the computer, as sitting for very long periods of time, according to latest research, can be as bad for you as smoking.

4. Glute bridges – 10 to 15.

5. Planks - regular ones and side planks.

Are the above mentioned core exercises and drills, or my five daily exercises too much for you, because you hardly have any time for anything? Then do the very best exercise for tennis players: burpees. Getting stronger doing one exercise a day not needing a gym has never been easier, so follow Krista Stryker's reasons from her article, *Five Reasons to do Burpees Every Day*.

1. Burpees work the entire body.
2. You can do them anywhere, whether you are at home, or traveling.
3. They will make you stronger.
4. They boost endurance with no need of a treadmill.
5. Burpees are a great addition to any workout, as they are dynamic, fast-paced, and never boring.

Although this chapter is dense with information and gives the beginner, intermediate, and advanced tennis player and athlete a variety of workouts, I encourage you to select the workouts that best suit your body needs and your time. Pick and choose carefully making some drills your "go-to" plan for a stronger and healthier you. Be mindful of your abilities and listen to your body.

Key points:

1. **Use the core and conditioning exercises** to become a stronger, better, and faster tennis player.

2. Out of all these exercise, **create your own routine that works for you** and you can find time to do it.

3. **Start your morning with 20 push-ups and 20 sit-ups** like I do, and your lower back will thank you.

4. **Lunges and squats** are one of the best exercises for tennis players, so incorporate them as you walk around the house, the tennis court, etc.

5. **Plank** as often as you can while watching TV, sitting around the house, etc.

6. **Do burpees on a weekly basis** to help with the explosiveness on the court.

7. **Be proactive!** Don't wait to get injured and then think about getting your body stronger.

8. **Extend your tennis longevity** by investing a few minutes daily in doing various exercises.

9. **Do not procrastinate and put off the exercises** with the excuse that you are playing a lot of tennis. Even one minute of squats and lunges will pay huge dividends keeping your knees strong, which I have learned the hard way through running.

10. Work to be **the strongest and fastest YOU!**

Disclaimer: I am not a trained professional in physical therapy or athletic training, but I have compiled these exercises from my own training by being on the college tennis team and from consulting various websites. Build up your strength and proceed at your own pace and athletic abilities. Consulting a physician is always good practice before you begin any rigorous exercise regimen.

CHAPTER SIX

Cross Training and Conditioning

"Tennis takes care of everything. It requires agility and quickness to get to the ball, core strength to get power into your shots and stamina to last for an entire match. In addition to toning your arms and shoulders, it's a total body workout for your legs and abs, and works your heart and core unlike any other sport."

Samantha Stosur

In one of the Grand Slam tournaments that I won in the 4.0 singles, I received a long sleeve T-shirt with the message *Tennis is life* emblazoned on the front. This has become my mantra. Because tennis gives us so much joy, balance, coordination, inner peace, and the ability to live in the moment, staying injury free is paramount to playing our best tennis. More importantly, if your goal is to play tennis all the way to 100 like me, cross-training and staying fit is essential to a lifetime of chasing the fuzzy yellow ball.

Here are a few ways to cross-train. Depending on your age and physical abilities, you can choose one or two exercises that will compliment and strengthen your tennis game.

Walking

Walking is what great tennis players do on the court. According to Jose Higueras, "tennis is a movement sport that requires efficient and effective footwork patterns as well as unbelievable balance. Great players have unbelievable rhythm with their feet."

Moving to balls on the tennis court is about putting one foot in front of the other, or "walking." The movement starts off with a good split-step, then the player flares the inside foot out in the direction he is moving, takes a strong crossover step, and by the third step he is loaded and ready to hit the ball from the singles sideline.

This is a perfect example of rhythmic footwork. Players should look to move in sequences of three steps. The best players in the world do not take one more step than is needed when moving to set up for a ball. Time is a gift you give to your opponent. It is a product of your movement, and the goal is to take time away from your opponent. Fewer, bigger steps, instead of more, smaller steps, will create greater efficiency, which will lead to creating more time for you on the court. In Spain, you hear coaches saying to the players, "camina, camina, camina," "walk, walk, walk."

Running

I started to run in March of 2015 after one of my friends showed me her running program *Strava* on her iPhone and went on passionately about her newfound love of running. I also decided to run to increase my stamina and do a different sport on the days I didn't play tennis. Try to walk, run, or bike to most places that are close to you, and you will feel so much better and fitter. Strive for more distance every day and combine at least two types of exercises. For me, it is running and hiking, biking and tennis, and running and Pilates/Yoga. It is amazing what a difference it made in my body, soul and mind. I also recommend jogging or running about two-three times a week for no longer than 5 miles the days when you are not playing tennis. This is so beneficial for your endurance and will increase your agility, footwork, speed, and mobility on the court.

For more ideas on running, feel free to subscribe to my running blog: www.runningforrealestate.com.

With tennis, our brains are constantly engaged and challenged to find new solutions and strategies to win the match. When we run, we simply allow our minds to relax and let go. To me, running is a meditation in motion. My focus is not on winning the next point, but on controlling my breath, as well as enjoying the shallow breathing and the calmness that running brings to the whole body. During my runs, the "thinking caps," so to speak, are of no use, as I strive to reach that inner peace and quietude combined with the runner's high.

Additionally, when we run, we increase our endurance level and prepare for tough and physically challenging matches. This preparation gives us an undeniable advantage over opponents who do not run as part of their routine. Running turns us into much stronger and more resilient tennis players. If running a half marathon or a marathon is your goal besides playing tennis, studies show that people who run marathons are more organized, disciplined, and efficient, which I totally believe.

During one of my runs, I asked myself: "How can we disrupt our complacency and satisfaction with things we do on all levels of our lives?" Answer: "By gently pushing ourselves to do more and requiring more of ourselves, as we are all perfectly capable of reaching higher professional, fitness, intellectual, and any other goals we set our minds on achieving."

Here are a few haikus, or shorter poems. Even though I did not strictly adhere to the exact haiku syllable count, they were inspired after various runs during my training for the first marathon, California International Marathon.

A Runner's Odyssey

Legs kick dust on the trail

mind churns ideas and thoughts

body bolts and jolts.

Runner's shoes

The shoes yoga mat insole

soft and airy cushions

life's fears of annihilation.

Of Shoes and Soles

The runner presides over

the tired soles of his shoes with

a calmed mind.

Yoga

I am sure you do not need much convincing about the tremendous physical and spiritual benefits of yoga. The word *yoga* means "union of mind, body, and spirit. It is the union between us and the intelligent cosmic spirit of creation. Yoga represents "The Oneness of all Things."

Yoga and tennis are both about letting go and being in the present moment. One of my yoga instructors at Family Fitness ended the class with this wise instruction: "With respect and gratitude, listen to your heart, your most valuable teacher."

All tennis players want to stay healthy for as long as possible. Practicing yoga at least once a week will help improve your flexibility and reduce your risk of getting injured. Recent scientific studies have shown that the regular practice of yoga also eliminates stress, improves breathing, digestion, blood pressure, and promotes losing weight.

Since our schedules are not always conducive to visiting a yoga studio before or after tennis, try doing these yoga poses at home or wherever you are before or after a match. These will help you maximize your flexibility and recovery. Here are a few yoga poses especially good for tennis players recommended in the August 2015 online *Yoga Journal*:

Crescent Lunge - stretches the hip flexors and chest. In this position, you stand with your right side near a wall or court fence. Step your right foot forward about 4 feet. Turn your torso slightly to the wall and place your right hand on it slightly behind you. Bend your right elbow to about 90 degrees, keeping it at shoulder height. Slowly bend your right knee until it's directly above your ankle as you turn your chest forward. You will feel a stretch in your right chest and the front of your left hip. Hold for 30–60 seconds. Repeat on the other side.

Cow Face Pose - (Do with tennis racket) is good for improving range of motion and stretching the rotator cuff. Grab the top of your racket with your right hand. Reach your right arm up over your shoulder and down your back. Place your left hand at the center of your lower back and grab the handle. The key is finding a position where you can relax the shoulders with a gentle stretch. If you're a right handed-player, hold for 1 minute; switch sides and hold for two minutes. If you're a lefty, hold for two minutes with right arm up; switch sides and hold for one minute.

Reclining side figure four - releases the outer hip, lower back, and IT Band, which runs from the outer hip to the outer knee. In this pose, lie on your back, bend your knees, and take your left ankle to your right knee, then take both legs to your right. Place the sole of your left foot on the floor as you send the left knee away from your head to feel a stretch through the left outer thigh and hip. Drop your left hip so your lower back relaxes. Hold for 1–2 minutes; switch sides.

Supine twist - good for stretching the muscles around the spine. Lie on your back, bend both knees, and take both legs to the right to rest on the floor or a pillow. Relax your back, hips, and then your entire body as you rest here. If you're a left-handed player, hold your knees to the right for about 2–3 minutes; switch sides and hold knees to the left for 1–2 minutes. Reverse the sequence if you're right-handed.

Tree pose - recommended by the United States Tennis Association. It is great for improving balance, as without proper balance and coordination, we cannot play our best tennis. In this pose, you simply bring the right leg to the side of your knee and bring your hands together in front of your heart, while standing in your pose for at least 30 seconds. After that, change legs, and repeat. Increase the time to one minute, as your balance gets better.

Besides practicing yoga to help stretch your body and prevent injuries, yoga is so quintessential in quieting the mind and reducing the negative chatter that most tennis players experience during matches. The controlled breathing technique called *pranayama* is a perfect tool to use to calm the mind and the nerves during tight matches. Yoga gives us a tremendous inner peace. Learning how to slow down your breathing will make you a better, stronger, and more composed tennis player. Being serene and focused in tight matches will turn you into a master of stability. It will help you perform on and off the court with a calm and undistracted mind.

Weights and Strengthening

As we know, tennis players need strong arms, legs, hips, and an even stronger core to be able to play tennis for life, because that's what we all want, right?

When it comes to weight lifting, Reed Stout, our American River College coach told us to work our muscles by using small three pound weights/barbells. You can start with ten sets of various lifting, such us lifting the weights over your head, doing lateral lifting, and bringing the arms in front. You can also combine balance and weights, and do two of my favorite and easy weight exercises:

Overhead push press - Stand on one leg (left or right), hold a dumbbell in each hand right above your shoulders with palms facing in toward your ears. Push the dumbbells straight up and come right back down, using your core to keep you balance. Do 15 of these, and if you have trouble balancing on one leg, try just touching your toe to the floor for a little stability.

Bicep curls - Stand on the opposite leg you did the overhead push press and hold a dumbbell in each hand straight down by your legs, palms facing forward. Curl both dumbbells up toward your shoulders, and then release them back down. Do 15 repetitions. I also highly recommend the lateral pull in the gym that works the upper body so well. Also when it comes to weights, you can do a ten minute workout at home, or you can use the gym to do a variety of exercises. Challenge yourself with heavier weights and develop the right routine for you, but wherever you choose to do it, remember that lifting weights two to three times a week will build your muscles and make you a stronger player.

Key points:

1. **Enjoy other sports besides tennis and cross train** to become better and stronger.

2. **Walking, running, yoga, weight lifting** are all great additions to making you a more well-rounded player.

3. **Stretching before and after matches** will keep you stronger and less likely to be injured.

4. **Run for increased stamina** and you will see your game go to the next level, as you will be winning longer matches.

5. **Mix core training**, such as push-ups and sit-ups **with weight lifting**.

6. **By practicing yoga** at least once a week, you will learn to breathe through your shots, as you hear so many coaches mention.

CHAPTER SEVEN

Breathing, Balance, and Staying Grounded

"Tennis is an art form, it is dance. It is how you shape time and space. It has a wonderful feeling."

Billie Jean King

One way to ace your tennis game is by mastering the two "B's": **"Breathing and Balance"**. The two concepts are intrinsically linked, while the third one, **"being grounded,"** is the foundation of these two.

When it comes to making great shots in tennis, breathing through your shots is essential. Most new players to the game will not understand one of the most important commands that tennis coaches make, which is "breathe through your shots." Whether you are a novice, or advanced player, I guarantee there have been many times you played a tight match and forgot to breathe through your shots. Breathing allows you to release tension, as well as be relaxed when hitting the ball, which is important to a successful stroke.

The calm, relaxed feeling you experience when breathing through your shots turns tennis into a spiritual experience.

Breathing on the court with purpose elicits joy, especially when doing something you like in an effortless manner. The same way we clear our minds when taking a cleansing breath, breathing through our shots nurtures a calm and peaceful mind on the court that will find solutions and strategies during tough matches. The result is clearer thinking and problem solving in tough matches.

Now that you are all convinced that breathing is essential to playing great tennis, let's explore some ways to incorporate breathing into your tennis game:

1. **Become aware of your breathing patterns**; most importantly, do not forget to breathe at all times.

2. **Inhale through the nose and exhale through the mouth** during all practice and competitive matches; especially during a long, intense match.

3. **Take a deep breath** when things do not go well on the court so that you can clear your mind and find renewed energy. It will help you turn your game around.

4. **Exhale as you hit the ball. Inhale after hitting the ball.**

5. **Learn to breathe smoothly and rhythmically** during aerobic training. This will become routine and enhance your breathing during tennis matches.

6. If grunting helps your breathing, as it helps me, do it. **Exhale with an audible, but controlled grunt**, one that is hopefully not too loud.

7. **Breathing is rhythmic**. Any time you feel you are not in sync on the court, it means you are not breathing properly, so the easy fix is to be aware of your breathing patterns and apply them well before you are out of breath and all tired.

8. **Controlled breathing** also equates calmness and composure. Breathe even more when you are behind and need to come back into the game.

9. **Proper breathing** builds confidence for better performance. Once I took up running and trained to run my first marathon in 2015, I understood how proper and correct breathing really increases my stamina and energy and who does not need more energy when playing tennis?

Have you ever wondered why balance is so important in life and sports? Do your friends and family always mention how they balance their lives to accomplish their goals and dreams? "It's all about balance," a phrase that continuously resurfaces and bounces high on people's lists like a well-executed topspin.

Before I started to take tennis seriously and had the drive to improve and become a better player, I used to look like a desperate gymnast walking on the beam of life and losing my footing. Balance used to be a foreign concept to me. I could have just as easily been learning a new language, because the terms associated with balance felt impossible to grasp. I soon learned that balance meant so much more than not falling flat on your face, so I have created a balance checklist that encompasses both mental and physical balance.

Physical Balance:

1. **Sure-footed balance**. Sure-footing, which simply means that your feet are confidently planted in the way you position them, dictates how your feet will navigate the court. For instance, when you want to hit a down the line two-handed backhand, your feet will face to the side of the court, not pointing cross court, whereas when you want to go cross court the tip of our feet are more diagonal pointing to the target. These positions begin with "sure-footed" balance.

2. **Balance with a wider stance**. A wider stance gives you more power and the ability to hit deeper balls with more pace and spin. The narrow stance that you use when you are rushed and don't have enough time to plant your feet wide, produce shorter shots and unforced errors.

3. **Balance = Being in the ready position**, ready to split-step, moving forward and backwards. This position with your knees bent, legs apart in a wider stance. Lower to the ground is crucial in tennis, as it allows you to cover a lot more court and be ready for the next shot.

4. **Being grounded** needs to feel as if your feet are one with the concrete, clay, or grass, plants rooted in the ground. It also means that your feet and legs will stay strong and help you generate the power on our shots together with a good hip rotation. In tennis, just like in life, you are trying to stay grounded as much as possible and accept the ephemeral nature of each point that, as John McEnroe remarked, "turns into poetry written on water." How many times have you

heard tennis coaches say: "Stay grounded! The power comes from your legs. Don't jump, reach, or lean, or you'll miss your shot!" "What is this guy talking about?" I asked myself when I first started to take tennis lessons as a self-rated 3.5 player. "What's wrong with a little jumping?" I continued my personal monologue. As my desire to improve my tennis game grew stronger, I became more aware of my hops and leaps, so I worked on moving more efficiently and staying grounded.

5. **More balance and ease**. When you play with ease and balance, your game is endowed with focus, clarity, superior execution, and more enjoyment on the court, as your shots are effortless and follow your lead. The player who exemplifies the most ease in his game is Roger Federer, of course. His composed movement is exemplified by the way he glides and paints the tennis court with his strokes like an artist. He doesn't seem to break a sweat and is one with the ball and the court. For him, tennis is such a labor of love, because he plays it rhythmically with relaxed muscles and upper body. Letting your arms relax will help you drive the ball deeper and conserve energy. We all have a lot to learn from the master of tennis. Strive to banish tightness from your game and welcome ease.

Mental Balance:

1. **Inner peace**, or being in charge of the mute button of your tennis remote control clears you mind and increases focus when striking the ball. When you silence any negative

thoughts that arise, you feel peaceful and confident that you can win matches. When you are peaceful in tight situations, such as tie-breaks, you will make smarter decisions on the court. Inner peace removes the mental static that interferes with good stroke choice, consistency and solid tennis that can draw errors from your opponent. You will develop a clear mind and a clear vision of what you need to do on the tennis court.

2. **Harmony** is achieving a perfect balance between your inner thoughts and outer reactions. Controlling the chatter is critical to physical response. Your task is to overcome any negativity, doubt, or fear. When thoughts are focused on physical movement and both are synchronized, performance levels improve and you will be more victorious on the court and off the court.

3. **Composure**. According to Lao Tzu, one of my favorite philosophers and Zen masters, composure is "the ruler of instability." I recommend reading his book, Tao Te Ching and applying its tremendous wisdom to your tennis game, and more importantly, to life. When you learn to stay composed and not be bothered by any external circumstances, such as noises, cheering, and loud people standing close to your court during playoff matches, districts, etc., you rule over your emotions and are successful in the execution of your best shots on the tennis court.

4. **Being grounded mentally and psychologically**. Besides the physical aspect, being grounded is equally important psychologically. When your mind is focused and not on an

emotional roller coaster, your thoughts are controlled and become one with the shot.

5. **Positive thinking and visualization**. Visualize yourself winning, coming back from behind, or simply planning where to place the ball on the court. Players of all skill level use visualization before, during, and after matches as a positive and "can do" reinforcement. Imagine yourself holding up the trophy when playing in tournaments, or just visualize the happy faces of your team mates after you had won a tough match that secured the win for your team. Be creative and find that image that will mentally propel your tennis game and help you play better and more focused tennis.

Now that we understand how important physical and mental balance is, let's analyze how various steps contribute to being grounded on the court and to developing modern-day footwork:

1. **The Walking Stance** - This movement requires just a small step to move into the court and hit a penetrating shot. Moving forward not upward equates more power and helps put weight behind the ball. In addition, by using a walking step, it is easier to move in any direction quickly and efficiently.

2. **The Cross Step** - A movement even more efficient than the walking stance, as you cross your foot over to hit a ball, but still remain in balance.

3. **The Karaoke Step** - (bringing one leg behind the other) A step perfect for transitioning forward into the court. It is

quite helpful to chip and charge the ball when hitting a slice backhand or forehand.

4. **The Hopping Stance** - Even though it sounds the opposite of being grounded, this step is good for players who are less flexible and are used more with a neutral stance.

Key points:

1. Tennis is all about **good posture and balance**. Stay grounded and hit your shots with ease and confidence.

2. **Being grounded and having controlled thoughts** will elevate your tennis game and will reduce your frustrations.

3. **Apply good breathing to your game**. When we forget to breathe through our shots, we will either miss, or make poor quality shots. Some people are better than others at breathing through their shots. If you are like me, forgetting to breathe, and needing to get CPR on the court, (as one of my coaches joked with me), then use a soft grunt or noise to help you. It will make a difference, especially in a long match.

4. Use tennis and its repetitive shots to bring out **the inner peace and joy**.

5. With tennis, just as in life, you need to prepared at all times and be in your **ready position** by judging the ball correctly and turning your shoulders.

6. **Be an artist** with your tennis rackets and be fluid with your strokes.

CHAPTER EIGHT

Speed and Split Steps

"Speed in tennis is a strange mixture of intuition, guesswork, footwork and hair-trigger reflexes. Many of the players famed for quickness on court would finish dead last in a field of schoolgirls in a race over any distance more than ten yards."

Eugene Scott

Every time I hear my coach remind me about splitting steps, I inevitably think of splitting hairs. Although in life we think deeply about solving a problem and tend to split hairs, in tennis, it is mainly a quick preparation for our next shot; whether it is the forehand, or the backhand. The split-step in tennis is the quick stop and go momentum that will help us position and attack the ball for our next big shot. In the beginning, I tried to envision this split-step many times, rolling it around my mind like a loose hair lock, but when it came to applying it on the court, I ended up jumping, hopping, hobbling, and stumbling.

"Dang! How could I split-step and still be standing on the court?" I asked myself confused. "What if the feet split and go in opposite directions?"

I understood that I had to widen my stance (feet apart), lower my body to the ground, and be balanced. Yet, to me, split-stepping was an extra step that I needed to take, when I was only interested in running and chasing ball after ball.

"You're too quick and you overrun the ball," a few of my coaches told me. "Always do your split-steps and be ready to hit your forehand or backhand. Think of it as a quick stop followed by a well-timed explosion on the court," one of the coaches told me. Even though I nodded in agreement, my mind was already splitting visually before my feet reacted.

After experimenting with running into the ball, as if it were an old friend, and consequently missing my volleys, I started to force myself to just stop so I could be ready for the next shot. Once I understood that my stopping needed to be smoother and that the split-step was pretty much synonymous with the split-second, practicing the split-step doing serve and volleys in doubles and in singles, was much easier. I started to be nimble on my feet and split-stepping became smoother. What I liked most about my new move on the court was the end result. I was sticking my volleys and finishing points with ease and grace. With everything new, the most important thing is to allow yourself to learn and be frustrated in the beginning. It is only through this learning process that your mind will crystallize the concept and commit it to memory. The new technique will soon become part of your tennis game.

Although the most important time to split-step is when we approach the net to make strong volleys, split stepping is very helpful when preparing to return serve. As the server tosses the ball into the air, a split step will ready us for the return so we can quickly move left or right. This can also be applied to positioning for most shots we hit on the court. That "split-second" step will help execute a quicker response to hit a winning forehand or backhand shot.

Key points about split steps:

1. **Never overrun** the ball.

2. **Make a quick stop** by the service line when moving forward.

3. After the quick stop, **control your feet** and be ready to go left or right.

4. **Make your split-step fluid** almost like a dance step.

5. **The more you practice it**, the more natural and effortless it will become.

6. **Split-step** when you prepare to return serves right when the player tosses the ball. Your returns will be stronger.

7. **Split-step when you serve and volley**, as you will be in balance and ready to stick your volleys or overheads.

8. **Split-step when hitting volleys** so that you can easily switch direction and hit forehands or backhands.

9. View the split-step as **the short pause, the "comma of tennis,"** so to speak that will allow you to hit the ball in balance.

10. **Be quick with your split-steps**, incorporate them into your game, and watch your game improve.

CHAPTER NINE

The Zen of Tennis

"Tennis is a perfect combination of violent action taking place in an atmosphere of tranquility."

Billie Jean King

There are a number of books written about the Zen of Tennis. All have one thing in common: composure! When people refer to Zen, they tend to think of deep meditation, focus, sitting meditation, and concentration, which are all indeed part of Zen, but when applied to tennis, it simply means **Carmen's "three C's of Zen": a cool, calm, and composed** mind that will separate a mediocre player from an exceptional player. When you practice and incorporate "the three Cs of Zen," you collect the "coolness, calmness, and composure" into your tennis bag of tricks and you simply become mentally stronger, less anxious, less worried about the next point, and more successful on and off the tennis court.

I never thought that I would be interested in learning as much as possible about Zen just to become a better and mentally strong tennis player, but I still remember one day in late winter when I met a tennis player who would later become my friend. Tamra was new on our 4.00 USTA tennis team and our captain wanted us to play singles against each other to know how to arrange her line-up. After exchanging a few balls and playing against Tamra, a sudden calmness took over me. It was as if her tranquil way of hitting the tennis ball impacted the way I played. Even my reaction to unforced errors became more composed. Since competing against players who got angry and upset with themselves and their opponents was a normal experience, meeting and observing Tamra's contained, calm, peaceful, and content demeanor on the court made me experience the "Ohm" of tennis, the ultimate Zen.

The ultimate Zen is **wise mindfulness**. It is reducing a storm to a mere, fine rain. This gives us focus to observe what works for a productive outcome and what is nonproductive. During my match, this meant smiling. Having noticed how Tamra smiled whether hitting the ball out or making the most amazing winning shot, made me feel part of the other side of tennis that is serene, tranquil, and calm.

At the end of our very long match, I felt that I needed to reach out to the latent Zen in me that gave me more confidence and the composure to execute smart and effective shots under pressure. Zen was the peace within my soul that once discovered, I could access it again and again. Zen had drowned out all the surrounding noises and voices, as well as the self-doubting voices inside my head. It helped me have a more relaxed attitude and play better tennis, especially in tight matches. Tight matches require a higher level of concentration where players need to resort to more strategy, more consistency and aggression at the right moment. The result should be a keen sense of when to sneak up to the net and execute a winning shot.

Another key Zen element that applies to tennis is the **equanimity of our minds**. When we apply Zen to tennis, we do not get upset about a poor shot or bad decision, and we do not get over excited about a terrific shot we made. With equanimity comes tremendous balance inside our minds and souls that requires the concentration and focus of a gymnast doing cartwheels on the balance beam. Rash decisions, raw emotions, venting, and anger are all tossed aside by the voice of reason that prevails over any kind of impulsive behavior.

Besides developing strong equanimity that keeps us in perfect balance in all kind of situations, we need to become **more responsive** to things that happen on and off the court, which is why being **pro-active vs. reactive** is so critical. On the one hand, when we merely respond and react to what is happening in life and on the tennis court, we put ourselves in a precarious situation, as we are too rushed to understand the consequences of our actions. On the other hand, when we make every effort possible to be pro-active by taking the ball early, as well as anticipating our opponents' shots, patterns, and intentions, we elevate the way we play tennis and feel more balanced. Being pro-active also allows us to come up with a game plan early on in the match.

I remember playing in a 4.5 tournament at Johnson Ranch in 2013 that I won. I was still ranked as a 4.0, but that year I had decided to play up. The first match I played against a player from the Bay Area who had a pretty weak backhand and an unimpressive topspin that she only hit cross-court. The weaker backhand became evident to me during warm-up, but the cross-court topspin I noticed after one game, so I immediately set out to be pro-active and position myself cross court to execute my signature shot: the down the line sliced forehand. I beat her easily in straight sets and felt great about disabling her game by noticing right away what her patterns were. When we are proactive, we are in control of our shots, emotions, and outcomes.

Control, a key component of our physical and mental game, is one of the most important words in tennis. When you play any match, either for fun or practice, your main goal and focus should be to take the control away from your opponent in order to reposition yourself on the court and execute your winning strategy. Control is the opposite of being reactive, which not only means that you are faster on your feet to dictate the match, but you are also thinking quickly and are ahead of your opponent by formulating an early game plan as soon as you step on the court. Shots made early in the match establish which player will dominate. When you execute winning shots and show your opponent that you're not just running down balls and yourself into the ground, you become a threatening opponent. Therefore, mental control leads to physical control, as you are focused on taking charge of the ball, but are also prepared to let go of the things that are out of your control, such as the demeanor of your opponent, one bad call, the loud spectators, the sun, the wind, and other distractions. Being in control of your body and mind is why Zen is important to tennis and why we need to apply more Zen to our lives.

Zen can help shift your focus from the importance of the outcome of the match to the greater goal of evolving as an athlete and a human being. Michael Jordan was a master at this. His main goal in life was the pursuit of total excellence. He constantly worked to turn his weaknesses into strengths. Tim Grover, Michael Jordan's personal trainer for fifteen years, recalls: "Michael's mindset was unique...he always felt someone else was going to outwork him. He had a big thing where he'd say, *'I'm going to turn my weaknesses into strengths.'* Every year there was evolution in his game. There was something he added; whether there was a new shot, or a new move."

Using the Zen approach and rules, you can become a focused tennis player who understands that winning, performing well, and feeling confident are very important, but only when they are tied with the goal of becoming something new, different, and even more exciting, the better version of yourself, which is easier to control than the outcome of a match.

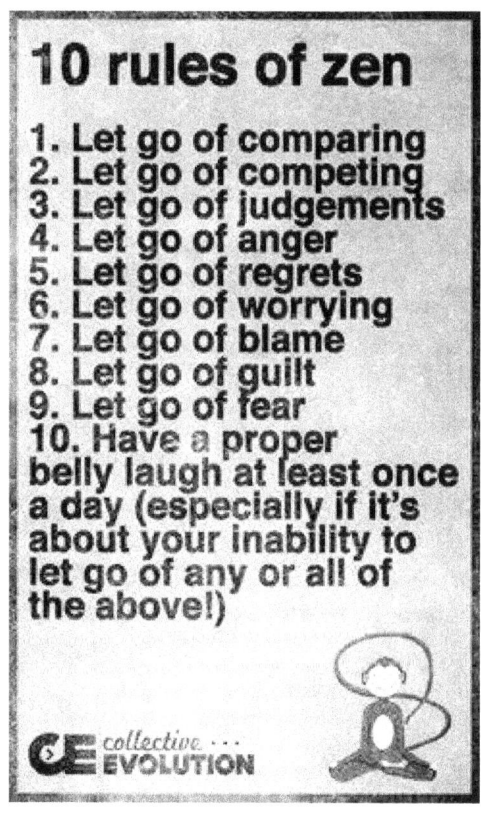

Key points:

1. Harness the Zen in you by **being mindful and purposeful**.

2. Make Carmen's three "C"s, being **cool, calm, and composed** part of your tennis game every time you step on the tennis court.

3. **Focus on the bigger picture** of becoming the best version of yourself instead of the immediate winning of a match.

4. **Find a peaceful corner** within your heart and mind and play with a Zen-like attitude.

5. **Learn to raise your focus, concentration, and determination** in key points and tight matches and winning will follow.

6. **Learn to accept external noises**, people talking, loud cheering, etc., and play with concentration and composure by accessing your inner peace and voiding the outer world.

7. **Harness the positive and reject any negative thoughts** that want to resurface during a tough match.

8. Instead of being focused on the competing, comparing, and judging, **learn to be the best you can be** by constantly challenging yourself.

9. Learn to **tap into your inner peace at all times**, by controlling the chatter, instead of letting your mind race.

10. **Play with composure** and relish the joy of hitting the ball.

11. **Be purposeful and mindful** with every shot, every move, and every point.

12. **Do not dwell on the past!** Once you have missed your shot, acknowledge your mistake, and move on to a better shot.

CHAPTER TEN

Mental Focus and Concentration

"The mind is your greatest weapon, the greatest club in your bag."

Golf Pro Steve Elkington

The connection between mental focus, concentration, and determination in tight tennis matches is the pivotal link between winning and losing a match. Some of my close wins demonstrate this importance where every point was critical, such as one match score of 7-6, 7-5. It felt so good to walk off the court with my victory! In the beginning, I did not understand why I won the close match and my opponent lost, but as more control and understanding of my tennis game evolved, I realized determination was key. Focus, composure, and execution allow you to work harder and smarter for every tie-break point. Speaking of tie-breaks, they used to be my worst nightmare. I often lost them and was petrified when we entered into a "tie-break."

As tie-breaks continued to hamper my spirit, a vision came to mind. At the end of the court was a throne. Above the velvety seat was inscribed in gold: *"Here sits Carmen, the Tie-Break Queen."* That changed my mental perspective on tie-breakers.

I wanted the crown. From that moment on, as a tie-break began, my subconscious would utter softly: "Carmen, remember? You are the tie-break queen!" The phrase alone turned my aggressive tennis on. It was evident that in order to win tie-breaks, a more aggressive attitude was necessary. I needed to attack at the right moment, as well as go to the net in key moments when my opponent least expected in order to win crucial points.

Besides playing really poised and focused tennis during tie-breaks, we need to use our mental concentration in two key situations:

1. When closing a match.

2. When we need to come back from being down.

I am sure we all have stories of matches we lost when initially we were leading 5-0. The biggest mistake players make when leading by a lot is relaxing and not playing with the same intensity that got them to that big lead. Another big mistake is taking your opponent for granted, saying to yourself too soon: "I got this." The cure to this problem: playing each tennis point with passion, intensity, and desire to close, as well as the humility to appreciate that your opponent might figure out a strategy and turn her game on anytime.

This is equally important in reverse. You are down 1-5, and your opponent thinks he/she has got you. To come back and win the set, you will need to deploy true grit, determination, full mental focus, a simple strategy that will work for that situation, and the "I can totally do this" attitude.

My most memorable comeback happened during a key match that I needed to win for my team. My opponent was familiar, so one of my plans was to attack her weaker backhand and try to win that way.

I started the match with great confidence, maybe too much of it, and quickly found myself in a deep hole. The score was 1-5 in my opponent's favor. At that moment, a light switch went off and I started to relax. By pure accident, an angle-slice forehand ripped from my racquet to my opponent who didn't even move her feet to the ball. I won the point. It occurred to me that her backhand was on fire that day and she was demolishing me with it. A new strategy emerged in my mind. These strategies helped me win the match and could work for you in future matches.

As part of my strategy, I made the conscious decision not to let go of the first set and just fight my way back. Instead of thinking just do it in three sets, I wanted to do it in two. I had to create a mental plan of attack and stick to it. My main focus was on hitting low slices to her forehand, taking her wide, so that I could open the backhand for a winner down the line. Here's the rest of my plan I quickly came up with during my match:

1. Play each point as if it were the last one.

2. Run like crazy on the court, chasing every single ball and trying to hit it deep to my opponent.

3. Instead of focusing on hitting a winner too soon, concentrate on the target and location of the shot.

4. Raise my confidence.

5. Believe in myself.

6. Never doubt I can win.

7. After being down 1-5 in the first set, I came back to not only win the first set, but the match 6-2 in the second set.

To me, coming up with the solution and the game plan felt natural, as I have played hundreds of matches and learned to think fast on the court, but if you are newer to the game or are still working on your mental strategies, here are a few ways to improve your mental toughness and ability to come up with a plan of attack. Apply these ideas during your practice matches and find a partner who plays at a similar level like you and wants to improve her mental game.

1. **Practice tie breaks** at the end of each practice match. Play one seven-point tie break and one ten-point tie break.

2. **Start your match being 5-1 up**. Work to close the match.

3. **Start your match being 1-5 down**. Work to come back and even win that set after you have come up with your strategic plan of attack and stick to it.

4. Practice **playing games with scores, such as 40-15, 15-40, 30-0, 0-40**, and so on that will make you play smarter, more aggressively, and improve your mental toughness.

5. **Practice serve and volley every time you are up 40-0,** as you have nothing to lose and that will make you more comfortable doing this during a competitive match.

6. Have a third friend sitting by the court make a lot of noise and be distracting so that you **learn to play with distractions**.

7. **Learn when to stick with your plan and learn when to be flexible** and come up with a different plan of attack and execution based on what's going on the court.

8. **Force yourself to attack more than defend** by being the first to control the point.

9. **Learn to stay in defensive mode for one or two shots**, after which look to attack again and take control of the point.

10. **Be analytical with your game and realistic**. Understand your strengths and weaknesses and be willing to make changes to your game.

Key points:

1. Develop the ability to **micro-manage the situation** by controlling each point a time.

2. Bring over the **strategies** used during the previous set that were successful before the tie-break started.

3. Each point is needed to win. **Staying in the moment** is key.

4. **Don't worry** about the last point.

5. **Don't rush**. Take your time to execute the shots.

6. **Quick assessment** of each point, without dwelling on anything that went wrong. Think about the next point.

7. **Have the drive to close** and make a tight tie-break situation a little loose and even relaxing.

8. **Follow your instincts**.

9. **Use mantras**, such as "you're the tie-break queen," "dig deep," "believe in yourself," etc.

10. **Stick to your plan** and do no change your mind when deciding upon a certain shot.

CHAPTER ELEVEN

Play Loose and Relaxed - Serve It Up!

"Life is like a game of tennis: the player who serves well, rarely loses."

Unknown

In 2013, while taking a once-a-week tennis lesson, there was a player taking a lesson before me that focused completely on practicing her serve. She was driven to develop the best serve she could for her ability. It seemed like she was obsessed when she should have concentrated a little more on other areas of her game. Yet, her quest for a great serve was not frivolous considering the only shot we control in tennis is our serve. If you have a strong serve with variety, such as flat, kick serve, topspin, and slice serve, you can simply control the outcome of many games when serving, while your opponent can only react to the kind of serve you produce.

Besides being confident in your serve, you have time to control your emotions and your motions. Your arm assumes the characteristics of a noodle; loose, yet strong at the same time. It can whip and snap the ball as you serve producing more power and executing a serve that will win more points. The secret to serving is constant work to improve your relaxed motions. Tightness is the enemy to serving. Fluidity, on the other hand, is paramount to serving with depth, speed, and pace.

Many shots in tennis are about releasing, executing with a relaxed upper body for serves and upper arm for ground strokes. Yet, finding that joy of relaxed execution is not as easy as it is for young players, such as my 10-year-old son, Alex. One summer day, after Alex finished his two-hour tennis class at Arden Hills Academy, I asked him how tennis was, and he replied: "I unleashed the serve today and even made some Aces."

"How did you do that?" I asked him.

"You just release it," he replied.

Kids don't over think and complicate matters like many adults. We can learn so much from their pure enjoyment and boldness.

As a self-taught player, serving has always been a difficult task to master. I used to jump and hop like a bunny, and my arm and upper body were definitely not relaxed. After taking a few tennis lessons, I understood that a more powerful serve happened when I planted my feet and stop the jumping craziness. Only after I played on the American River College team, I learned how to serve properly, and my serve became more of a weapon than a liability. I also learned to develop the flat, topspin, kick, and slice serves. This confidence has resulted in me choosing to serve when winning the toss.

If you are asking yourself: "How do I develop a great serve?" Practice and repetition yield confidence, especially in tight matches where your serve is critical. Take a few lessons, read tennis articles, and watch YouTube videos. Here are a few recommendations:

http://volleycam.com/tennis-serve-training/

https://www.youtube.com/watch?v=ef1ZeWAA2gE

http://www.active.com/tennis/articles/tennis-serve-training-tips-and-drills

I have met players with phenomenal serves who were diligent in developing their serve by practicing after watching these videos and applying the tips in the videos. Applied knowledge is vital to success in everything we do.

According to the author Dennis Van Der Meer of *7 Steps to a Perfect Serve* that appeared in the *Active.com* online magazine, there is always room for improvement when it comes to serving. In order to help readers detect their weakness when serving, Van Der Meer points out that we need to look at the following aspects of our serves:

- reliability of first serve
- pace generated
- effectiveness at hiding the direction of the serve
- depth consistency of serve
- effectiveness of serve
- proper execution of serving under pressure

Developing a reliable first serve will strengthen your ability to win your serving game and not be broken. Van Der Meer suggests using the following serving drill to help increase the accuracy of your serve. First, divide the service square into three equal sized areas. Then serve wide to the outside box, then the middle, and down the center line, or to the T. Make sure you can aim and serve successfully into each area before moving to the next.

Another component for serving well is rhythm. For instance, bouncing the ball three times before serving gets us into the flow and prevents us from speeding up our serve. Not rushing is part of having a great rhythm and serving with a live arm. A live arm will help generate a more affective serve. There are several components to developing a live arm: fluidity of motion, total looseness and flexibility resulting in an explosion of power, and stability at the point of contact. This will add more power to the serve by using a stable, but not stiff arm.

In addition to these concepts, I also learned more ways to serve well during my college training:

1. Start with a relaxed body and arm.

2. Bend the knees and tilt the body to create a heavy spin serve.

3. Bring the racket behind your shoulder.

4. Bring the elbow away from your body, as if you were elbowing someone. According to former top 100 ATP Jeff Salzenstein, this motion alone is huge. It can increase the speed of your serve by up to eight miles per hour.

5. Get the ball in front of your head.

6. Watch the ball's height in the air when serving.

7. Hit on top of the ball.

8. Pronate, which means snapping your wrist to the right, if you are a right-hand player.

9. Bring your serving arm around the body, as if wrapping yourself in a shawl.

10. Bring your body weight into the court.

Another great way to improve your serves is to work on your arm strength. When I trained with my ARC team, Coach Reed made us toss the ball from the service line all the way to the fence. Once we could hit the fence, we would move to the baseline and try to hit as hard as we could into the court. When I first started the drill, I realized how weak my arm and shoulders were. After doing this a few times, I got stronger and more confident in my upper body strength. Lifting 3-pound or 5-pound dumbbells about twice a week also improved my arm strength and made me less prone to injuries.

Key points:

1. **Improve your serve** by learning and practicing flat serves, topspins, kick, and slice serves.

2. Get a basket of balls and **practice serving** at least once a week. Be purposeful and mindful where you place the ball and what type of serve you are practicing.

3. Make sure you always allow **time to warm-up your serves** before every practice, league, or tournament match.

4. During matches, don't forget to **alternate your serve** after your opponent gets used to the serve.

5. **Notice what type of serve** brings you more results during matches. Hone that particular serve to develop its reliability.

6. **Learn to disguise** the location and the type of serve by developing a very consistent toss that can be applied to all type of serves.

7. When serving to close the game, set, or match, **clear your mind and calm your jittery body**.

8. **Do not think or worry about double faulting**, which is easier said than done; instead, focus on the location and type of serve you will do and release your arm with confidence.

9. **Practice, practice, and practice some more!** Positive results will emerge!

CHAPTER TWELVE

Embrace Change by Playing Singles and Doubles

"I feel my biggest contribution has been to get people to think more intelligently about the game."

Vic Braden

Just as we want to be well-rounded in life, we need to embrace change, be well-versed and all-around court players in tennis. When I first started to play tennis, I played singles exclusively. At first, I didn't even know how I hit the ball to create my slice. I was not pro-active. I played reactive tennis, as I constantly jumped around reaching and lunging for balls without having any sense of balance and coordination. The excitement of hitting the ball prevailed over any sense of purpose on the court.

After a few years of playing tennis against my husband, we discovered tournaments and leagues, where we tried to give our opponents our unconventional, crazy shots to win the match. Even though my husband had more tools in his tennis bag than me, I was a shrewd player with super ugly form that made other players roll their eyes in frustration and disappointment, thinking that there should be no way they lose to me. In those first years of tennis, guidance on the whole aspect of the game would have been helpful. Since I did not have any, I resorted to being a ball chaser. My goal was to keep the ball in the court for as long as possible, thus having super long rallies (one time I had a 50 ball rally that I won). Being a grinder yielded good results for me at the 3.5 level.

After two years, I moved up to the 4.0 level and started playing more competitive tennis. Due to the more intense matches and better players I played against, I knew that I needed to play smarter tennis. I also started to take lessons to undo the craziness of my game and to become a more consistent player.

One step at a time, the change in my tennis game happened this way:

1. I learned different ways to serve.
2. I switched my grip to a Continental from an Eastern when hitting my slices.
3. I started to learn topspin.
4. I became more focused and more interested in playing with a purpose.

Having a purpose and an attainable goal in tennis is just like in life: you embrace change and implement strategies that will help you become successful. Changing and undoing the incorrect form I had developed on my own was harder than learning tennis from zero. Therefore, I had to pay more attention to my form, to the way I held the racket, and how to hit the ball to create spin, and so on.

I owe a big thank you to my very first coach Betsy Kessing who teaches at Arden Park in Sacramento. When she first met me, she thought I was hopeless and would resist change, until she realized that I was seriously interested in changing my game and leaving the mediocre player behind in order to climb up the tennis ranking and infuse meaning and purpose to my tennis game. She was encouraging and helped me make the biggest adjustment to my game by changing my grip from an Eastern to a Continental one for my slices. Once I changed the grip, my slices, or my signature shot, were even meaner driving my topspin opponents crazy. Betsy also taught me all the various type of serves in just one session. I learned to do the flat, topspin, slice, and kick serve, but it took me many years after that to make the serve stronger.

Every coach I took lessons from made quintessential changes to my game and loved that I was like a sponge, learned fast, and most importantly, I was willing to change. With three things guaranteed in life: death, taxes, and change, you might as well fully embrace the last one. You will reap the benefits in time.

As a pure singles player in my first years of playing tennis, change was not easy, as it affected my consistency. However, once I realized that changing and tweaking something in my game will trigger a few more mistakes in the beginning, I surfed on top of the frothy wave until the change became organic to my game and I could execute my shots better than before.

After taking lessons from at least six tennis pros, I developed a decent arsenal of meaner slices, as most of my friends called them, high topspins, better and stronger backhand, and sharper volleys. I started to play singles with purpose. For instance, if my opponents handled my slice well, I would deploy topspin lobs and move in to the net, especially after attacking their backhand. Being cognizant of what shots to apply on the court really pays off in singles, as you are on your own with no partner to guide you. Doing different things on the court, such as hitting softer and harder balls, as well as sneaking to the net after a skipping slice or a high topspin to your opponent's backhand helps you play the best game against a particular opponent, which is why many players tell me I am a smart player. It has been beneficial to keep notes on tough players, so I can adjust my game in the future. The notes may help me find ways to adjust my game and deploy a different strategy that is more conducive to winning that match. The strategies I used in singles, soon became very effective in doubles, as not many doubles players play singles. Additionally, the consistency that helped me win in singles was a big weapon in doubles.

The most notable change in my game that doubles matches provided was my comfort level at the net. Although coming to the net was never part of my game until I started to play doubles, now I like coming to net and having fun putting volleys and overheads away, after I have set myself up with a good, deep shot.

In the beginning, doubles seemed like a chess game to me with a lot of thinking involved as to the strategy applied to each point. I also had to learn to switch sides with my partner, poaching, moving around in the service box, and, most importantly, learning to read the trajectory of the ball. As opposed to playing singles, when you have to cover the entire court and scramble for every ball, in doubles, it is all about the right positioning, as well as applying a geometric thinking, placing the ball and using more angles to close the point, which is also true of singles.

After taking a few doubles clinic with various coaches, I became more comfortable playing doubles. I started to really enjoy poaching the ball as much as possible, leaving my side wide open for a down-the line winner from the opponent, but unless the opponent could make that winning shot at least three times, I would still continue to poach. Another thing about doubles is identifying target areas to force errors from your opponent. Even though we are trying to find the open space on the court as much as possible, learning to hit the ball at the other player's feet, right hip, and high over the opponent's shoulder on the backhand side will force errors and bring easy winning points.

Just as singles players who understand the ideal court positioning make good doubles players because of their consistency, doubles players make great singles players due to their good volleys, overheads, and their confidence to move to the net and close the point. Additionally, playing both singles and doubles improves your footwork, your court awareness, and overall improvement of your shot selection and execution.

Key points about playing singles:

1. **Great workout**, as you are the only one chasing all the balls.

2. **Taking responsibility for your own mistakes**, as there is no partner to blame.

3. **Strategizing on your own** and thinking fast on the court.

4. **Consistency**.

5. **Patience** is key when playing singles, more than doubles, as rallies can be long, and in most cases the most patient player wins.

6. **Trial and error**, meaning that sometimes you need to try something new that might work or not, but be prepared to take this risk.

7. **Good focus and concentration in key moments**, such as leading 5-4 and serving for the match, or being down 4-5 and trying to bring it to 5-5.

8. **Rhythmic breathing** is your best ally, or breathing through your shots to conserve energy.

9. If you are good at chasing balls down and don't mind playing a long match, **turn your singles match into a marathon**, and see who is fitter and can run and rally longer.

10. **Be willing to use different tools** if what you are doing is not working.

11. **Be willing to change** from one game or set to another; transform into a different player who is not afraid of trying something new when things don't work out on the court.

12. **Resist insanity**, or what Einstein called doing the same thing over and over and expecting different results. Instead, apply a new strategy that will make a difference, even though it might not always lead to a win, but will provide you with options every time you play singles.

13. **More court to work with** and place the ball away from your opponent.

14. **Come to the net** when you push your opponent deep.

15. **Practice different shots**, as your opponent has more court to cover. Not making the perfect volley will be more forgiving than in doubles.

16. **Play with joy and apply Zen** when things get tough.

17. **Be your own cheerleader**.

18. **Play grounded and humble**, which is my main mantra that I apply to tennis, especially singles.

Key points about playing doubles:

1. Playing doubles gives you the chance to **play the net more**, which turns you into a stronger and better singles player.

2. **You strategize more**, which helps you come up with more ideas, solutions, and thus diversifies your tennis game.

3. **You get to practice serve and volley more than in singles**, as you only have to cover half the court. This can benefit your singles game.

4. Playing doubles helps you **be aware of the ball at all times** and keeps on your toes, as the game moves faster and your reactions need to be quicker.

5. It will make you **play smarter**, as you need to adjust constantly to your opponents, as well as find solutions from one set to another.

6. **It will make you use different shots**, as the combination of topspin and slice will give your opponents trouble.

7. **It will make you a better communicator**, as talking to your partner is critical in doubles.

8. **It will make you step outside your comfort zone** and turn you into a team player, as in doubles you cannot win without your partner. You win and lose together.

9. **It will improve your overheads** and turn you into a confident singles player from the net.

10. Playing doubles will provide you with **double the fun**. Enjoy!

CHAPTER THIRTEEN

Expand Your Tennis Toolbox with a Variety of Shots and Strokes

"Tennis is like playing chess at 120 miles per hour."

Robin Williams

The 2015 U.S. Open was an eye opener for women's tennis due to the semi-final between Serena Williams and Roberta Vinci. That match showed us that power alone does not ensure a win. Vinci beat Serena in three sets using topspin and slice backhands, mixing volleys from the net with drop shots and overall smart tennis. Vinci also demonstrated that she could handle Serena's power shots and even redirected that power to turn the point around and win it.

The importance of learning different shots became clear when I started to play matches against 4.5 players. They seemed to have a lot more tools and tricks and could deploy whatever shot they needed against their various opponents. For instance, if someone handles your topspins so well that you mostly lose the one-on-one rallies, then change to a slice. Another option is to just slow down the balls so that you your opponent has to adjust footwork and the way she hits the ball. During a recent tournament my lefty opponent loved my sliced forehand, which is my best and infamous shot, as most players have little success handling it. As a result, I decided to change and mainly play a high loopy topspin to her backhand. Sure enough, I racked up points easily and won the match 7-5, 6-0. At the end of the match, she told me:

"I didn't know you were such a lobber!"

"Well, as you know, that's not my regular game, but I had to adapt, since you liked my slice and put those shots away so many times," I replied.

When you have a variety of shots, playing against an array of opponents becomes easier and more fun. You decide which tool would be effective to pull out of your tennis bag. Adapting to your opponent is the first step. Once you observe what your opponent likes or does not like, then you know which shot or strategy to apply to win the match.

In my case, my "go to" shot is the slice forehand and the two-handed backhand. When I need to deploy other shots, I use my topspin forehand lobs, which set me up to go to the net. The slice backhand changes the way the ball bounces, too, and can be used effectively as a "chip and charge" strategy.

The strength of having multiple shots means that you not only observe, adapt, and change the way you play depending on your opponent, but you also approach tennis intelligently. You constantly think on the court and evaluate what you need to do to come back from behind in a match, or to simply close a tight match. A repertoire of shots opens multiple opportunities to strategize your game. It makes you a more creative and crafty player as you constantly plot your game, take calculated risks, and use various strategies to help you play your best.

It is quite essential that you take risks employing your new shots in practice matches. It will ultimately become a routine shot that can be used competitively in future matches. Another way to apply a new shot you just learned is during an easier match where you can afford to be adventurous, while disrupting your comfort level.

After I played a tournament at Sutter Lawn, the tournament Director, Jason Johnson complimented me on my wicked forehand slice. He then asked me:

"Why don't you use the same type of spin on the other side?"

"Because I don't have it," I replied honestly.

"We can easily fix that," he said.

I was thrilled to have him teach me a two-handed slice backhand. It helped me win some easy points using it to drop shot or place deep shots. Variation is so important in tennis, as well as breaking up the pace of your opponent.

From 2010 until now, I took tennis lessons and realized that some tennis pros are not too keen on teaching slice. I started gravitating to coaches who appreciated backspin and did not try to tell me to stop using slice and mainly play topspin, because this is how modern tennis is played.

Having taken lessons from various pros has helped me learn different shots and strategies faster with less frustration and in a more dynamic way. Do not feel guilty working with different coaches. They all have their way of teaching which will give you a different perspective on your game while becoming a more confident player.

Key points:

1. **Diversify your game** by learning topspin and slice.

2. Assess your opponent's strengths and weaknesses and **apply the right strategy** or shot to increase your chances of winning.

3. **Take lessons from various pros** to learn different shots and strategies that you can use on the court.

4. When you're playing against stronger player, **take risks and do something different**.

5. **Approach tennis intelligently**, as if playing chess, and plot your next move to throw your opponent off.

6. **Be creative**.

7. **Be willing to change** and get out of your comfort zone.

8. When you are up 40-0, or 40-15, make it a habit to **try a new shot**, such as serve and volley, and see what happens.

9. **Vary your game** and use different speeds to disrupt your opponent's tennis game.

10. And last, but not least, **have fun playing and experimenting**.

CHAPTER FOURTEEN

Rackets and Strings

"I'll let the racket do the talking."

John McEnroe

When I first started to play tennis with my dear father back in Romania, there was no fretting over rackets. I only had one choice: the wooden racket that I could barely hold and lift. Nonetheless, I was ecstatic to get my first racket and so eager to learn how to play. Nowadays, with a myriad of choices in rackets, strings, and any accessory imaginable, we face a big dilemma as to what racket and strings to choose.

Multifilament strings are softer and add extra spin on the ball. However, when players complain of tennis elbow, we have to look at the racket and the strings. If the racket is too light, then the arm and elbow will receive the vibrations and they will hurt.

One time, my husband bought me a beautiful, but light tennis racket for Mother's Day. Unfortunately, playing with it was painful. I never thought it was the racket; instead, my focus was on my ripe age of 34. My friends even made fun of me! All I could think of was to write a poem about getting older, instead of making the connection between pain and playing with the wrong racket.

Getting Older and Stronger

A white hair - iridescent first slithers

among all the brown hairs,

but who has time to split hairs?

When feeling the invincibility and candor of

youth unfurled in the shape of butterfly pink and purple

carnival glasses matching flamboyant me!

I'll defeat old age and grayness with my slicing and dicing

of life, which is nothing but a tennis match served well.

But, then wait. A sharp pain down my elbow nags at me

Lately when I play tennis.

Our team captain says: "It's tennis elbow.

You'll have to nip it in the bud."

Rubbing my right arm, I reply:

"No, I think I'm just getting older and stronger."

"Life's not always a flaming grill," I continue my thoughts.

Plucking moonlight hairs.

This is why it was important to include a special chapter about racquet choices. Your racquet can have a great impact on both your game and your physical ability. Although a light racket is easier to maneuver and one can swing harder, there is not much power going into the ball. A heavier racket will help you hit harder and crush the ball. Playing with the wrong racket for your arm could really affect your game and even cause damage to your arm. Investing in a good racket that works for you is fundamental to maintaining a healthy, strong, arm. Playing with a heavier racket, using proper form, getting your muscles stronger by lifting weights a few times a week will make tennis more fun and help you win more matches.

When my husband and I first came to America and started to play tennis every week, we did not know what racket to buy and had no idea that light rackets would be bad for our tennis game and our elbows. My racket was a light 8 oz, and it wasn't until I started to take tennis lessons with tennis pro Milun Doskovic at Gold River Racket Club that he told me I was playing with "an old lady's racket," as he joked. I was in my early 30s, and according to my coach, I needed to go to Courtside and demo rackets ASAP, so that I can get a heavier racket that will help me learn good topspins and change my game. It was amazing that no other tennis pro took the time to point that out to me. It soon became clear how hard it was to take your game to the next level using the wrong tennis equipment.

After having tried a few rackets at Courtside, I settled on a Prince racket that was 9.2 oz, quite an improvement from my old 8 oz racket with a large head. I immediately started to play better and my arm pain went away. I was amazed at this simple solution. Since then, I share this information with players who appear to be using the wrong racquet, although the best way to know is to talk to a tennis pro and evaluate your entire game, your type of racket, your goals in tennis, and your willingness to change.

Whenever I play league and tournament matches, I still meet players who play with older type rackets that are too light for them, but some are not willing to change, or think that a heavier racket will make their arm hurt. Just because most players use heavier rackets nowadays, you still have to choose the right racket that works for you, as everybody is different. One recommendation that worked for me might not work for you, but trying rackets and doing your research will surely help.

After having played with the Prince racket for a few years, I needed one more change. In 2014, after I broke the strings of my racket during my lesson with coach Amine Khalid, I bought the Babolat Pure Drive, which weighs 10.6 oz. The year I bought my racket, most of the pros were using the same racket, so I felt good that I finally got the right racket. Once again, I was able to elevate my game and play better tennis than before with lots of practice and changes to my game.

In 2015, after having had the best tennis year ever with an outstanding record both in leagues and tournaments, I upgraded my Babolat Pure Drive racket and added some lead weights around the handle, which changed the weight to 11.2 oz. I could have just bought the new *Babolat Pure Strike* or even the 2016 *Pure Aero Babolat* (the racket weighs 11.3 oz and has a wider cross-string spacing and added string movement to enhance spin production, although it is not as good for touch shots), but, instead, I chose to go to Courtside Tennis to retrofit my racket, so that I could be prepared to play higher level tennis as a new 4.5 player.

It was important to include this chapter on choosing a good racquet, because of my long journey with rackets, which has impacted my overall game and physical ability on my trek from a 3.5 to 4.5 player. My tennis experience has been well worth it, and I hope that some of you will get higher rankings faster and with fewer explorations. Sharing what I have learned about tennis will hopefully, make your journey smoother and more fun.

Carmen's tips and key points for buying a new racket:

1. Demo good rackets at tennis stores. In Sacramento, we have Courtside Tennis. The people working there are very knowledgeable and will guide you in the right direction. Explore your area for a professional tennis shop and tell them your level of play. For instance, a 3.00 player has different needs than a 4.00 player. One needs more control, while the other player needs more power.

2. Try at least six different types of rackets, such as Babolat (I'm playing with a retrofitted Pure Drive, 11.2 oz Babolat, which I love!), Prince, Head, Wilson, Yonex, Wilson, etc.

3. Keep notes of your performance, feel, likes/dislikes when trying new rackets.

4. Try to start with the right racket from the beginning to reap more benefits and propel your tennis game faster.

5. Be aware that the strings on the demo rackets are quite basic, so you will play better when using the right strings.

6. Experiment with various strings depending on what you want to achieve on the court, whether is spin or control.

7. Once you found the best match, eventually you will need to buy the same racket so that you have two identical rackets in your tennis bag.

8. Really get to know your racket so that you can use it to your advantage in any match situation.

9. If you play about three times a week, you will need to change your strings every three months, whether they break or not. For players who only play once a week, you can get up to six months, but the best thing is to always check your strings, and if they are frayed, it is time to get new ones.

10. Remember you and your racket have to make the perfect duo, so team up wisely!

Tips and questions to ask yourself from *Tennis Magazine* (March/April 2014 edition) on choosing the right stick:

1. What am I searching for? This question is crucial when it comes to buying a new racket. It takes a lot of time and money to buy the right racket, so evaluate what your goals are, such as adding more spin to your shots, more pop, increasing the swing speed, etc.

2. How should I rate each frame? For instance, if your serve is your best shot and the new frame you are trying does not match that, then the frame is out of the question. Using a grading scale when trying new rackets will definitely help you narrow things down and buy the right racket.

3. Am I willing to put the old faithful aside? Even though you are not going to play as well with the test frame as your regular one, with little tweaks and small adjustments on your part, you will start playing well with your new racket and elevate your game, so be willing to work a little bit with the new frame, instead of doing demo after demo and not committing to making the change.

Key points:

1. **Invest in a good tennis racket** that works best for your game.

2. **Be willing to part away from your old racket** if you feel your game is stagnating.

3. **Change is good**. Do not be afraid to try new rackets and see if they can improve your game besides the things you are already doing.

4. **Lighter rackets allow you to swing faster**, but they do not allow you to hit harder. Playing with a heavier racket will make you hit harder and deeper with less effort and most likely less elbow pain; especially if you get your arm muscle stronger.

5. Do not use a certain type of racket because your favorite tennis player plays with that racket. Instead, **play with the racket that is right for you**.

6. Once you have the perfect racket that you like, **buy a second one exactly the same to have if you break strings** during matches.

7. **Experiment with rackets and strings** until you have found the perfect combination and formula for a better and happier tennis player.

CHAPTER FIFTEEN

Got Grips? Tennis and Life Grips

"Tennis points may be inspiring at the moment, but then the moment is gone. They're like poetry written on water."

John McEnroe

Tennis is an open door when experimenting with new grips. Using the Western, Eastern, Continental, or any variation of the grip, can produce radically different results with spin, pace, and placement. In the game of tennis, grip is paramount in the execution of the perfect point-getting shot. This diagram will explain more about the bevels of the racket, which are the best way to help players understand the various grips and how they are achieved.

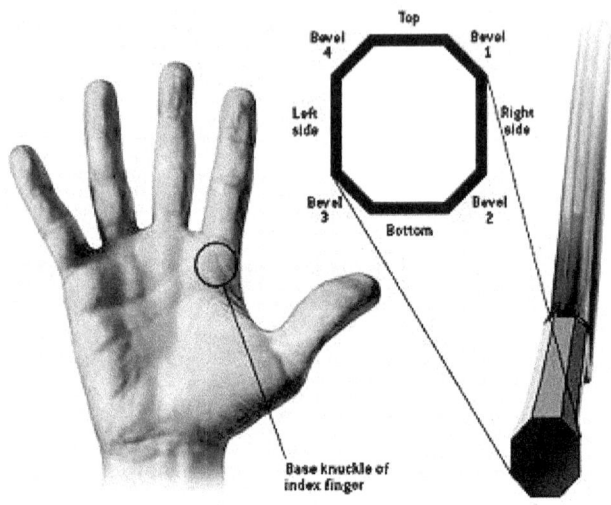

Since grips are so much about positioning your hand on the racket, I have come to understand them better not by analyzing the handle of my racket, but by examining the two most common grips. For instance, **the Continental Grip** is created by your base knuckle of your index finger on bevel 2 (the top-facing bevel on your eight-sided handle is 1), or as one of my coaches told me that the grip is the same as shaking someone's hand. The continental grip is the handshake grip that should be a firm, yet relaxed grip on life. "The continental grip is used primarily for serves, volleys, overheads, slices, and defensive shots," Jon Levey pointed out in his article *The Grip Guide* published in *The Tennis Magazine*.

How to Get the Continental Grip:
1. Hold the racket so the knuckle on your index finger that is closest to the palm of your hand is on Bevel 2.
2. The heel of your hand should just about rest on Bevel 2 at the end of the racket.
3. The "V" formed by your thumb and index finger should be on top of the racket, on Bevel 1.

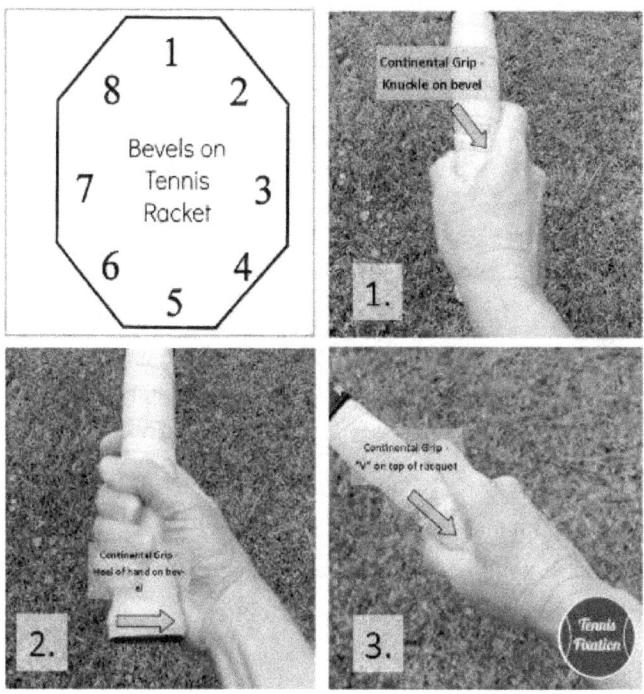

The **Eastern Forehand Grip** is considered the easiest grip to learn. It is simply achieved by moving your base knuckle of your index finger onto bevel 3. For "righties," you move clockwise from 2 to 8 when you look at the hands of a watch. Another way to find this grip easily is by picking up the racket from a table. With this grip, topspin is effective. Using this grip makes it easy to change to the continental grip for volleys and coming to the net. I use this grip for topspins because it was easy to learn and proved effective in my game.

The **Semi-Western Forehand Grip** was presented to me as the "frying pan grip," since it imitates picking up and holding our rackets as if we were flipping pancakes. Moving your index finger knuckle from the Eastern forehand to bevel 4 grip puts you in a semi-western grip. Most tennis pros encourage their students to use this position, as it is the prevalent grip for power baseliners on the pro tours.

The **Western Forehand Grip** requires you to shift your index-finger knuckle one more bevel clockwise (Counterclockwise for lefties) to bevel 5, which puts your knuckle on the very bottom of the grip and your palm almost completely under the racket, as Levey points out in his article. This grip generates a lot of spin, but it is quite inefficient when it comes to hitting low balls, as well as moving to the net, so most coaches steer players away from the Western grip.

The **Two-Handed Backhand Grip** is one of the most used grip for backhands, especially for players who do not have a good one-handed backhand. Once I changed to this grip when working on my backhand, my backhand became so much stronger, reliable, and more of a weapon than a liability. The most common way is to hold the racket in your dominant hand with a Continental grip. Take your other hand in a semi-Western forehand grip with the index knuckle on bevel 6.

Eastern Backhand Grip is accomplished when from a Continental grip, you shift your index-finger knuckle on bevel counterclockwise (clockwise for lefties) so that it is on the very top of the grip on bevel 1. This grip provides good stability especially for low shots, but it is not as effective against kick serves and shoulder level topspins.

Semi-Western Backhand Grip, just like the Western forehand grip, is not the preferred grip due to its difficulty and less versatility. Players who have a Western forehand grip use it, especially when rallying from the baseline, as some of the most powerful backhands are held with this grip. With this grip, the base knuckle of your index finger moves one bevel counter-clockwise (clockwise for lefties) from the Eastern backhand to bevel 8.

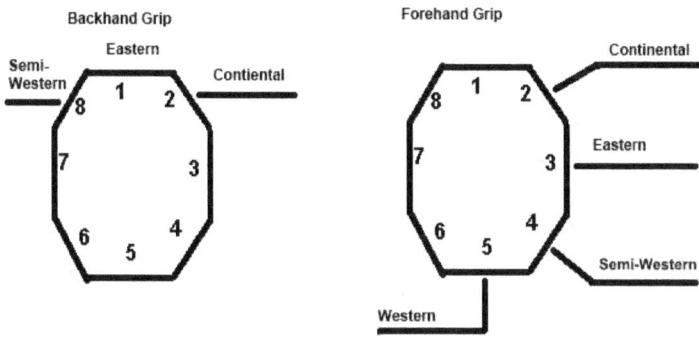

Being a self-taught player, I started to play tennis using an Eastern grip. After taking lessons from various coaches, as I felt that they all had something different and unique to teach me, I have learned to rely on the continental grip for my slice forehands and my two-handed backhand and to use the Eastern grip for my topspin forehands. Being aware of how you hit the ball when using a certain grip is acquiescing life, as you notice what works and what doesn't work; you adjust your perspective and look to change the things that no longer serve you with more productive and efficient goals and strategies. Grips are also our constant guides in tennis, as they are showing us the cause and effect on and off the tennis court.

Key points about tennis grips:

1. **A changed grip** gives you a different spin and perspective on things.

2. **Don't forget to change grips** when coming to the net, from an Eastern or semi-Western to Continental.

3. Allow yourself to **experiment with various grips**.

4. Allow yourself **to be uncomfortable when learning** a new grip.

5. Tennis and life are about adopting **more productive and efficient habits**.

6. You're tense and grip your racket too tightly; **remember to loosen up and relax**.

7. The Western grip is considered an extreme grip in tennis, because players who have this grip have consistency issues and trouble playing the net, so change it to a semi-Western, and **stop struggling**.

8. **A small shift in angle**, or the way you hold the racket gives you a different feel and perspective on tennis and life.

CHAPTER SIXTEEN

Eating a Balanced Diet - Proper Nutrition

"One should eat to live, not live to eat."

Molière

While training to run my first California International Marathon in 2015, I deepened my love and knowledge about nutrition. I ran my first marathon with a good time of 4:13:21, which gave me hope to keep training and try to qualify for Boston. I also realized that no matter how hard we train in tennis or running, without proper nutrition, we will break down and crash in long matches. To understand more about creating energy in my body through food, I loved reading articles about nutrition, as I learned something new every time. Although some think that tennis is a sport that doesn't require much running and agility if you just strike the ball hard and make your opponent move, taking your game to the next level requires vigorous movement which comes from eating a balanced diet, or lots of vitamin F, which stands for real food.

In my case, most of my friends call me the "energizer bunny", as I have tremendous energy on and off the court and love playing long matches. However, the main difference in my stamina came in 2012 when I decided to become *pesco-vegan*. The pesco-vegan diet follows the vegan diet, meaning no dairy products, no meat, no eggs, but adds seafood and wild fish, which are good sources of Omega-3s and are great for brain function. In less than a month, after I changed my diet, my energy level doubled and I felt twenty years younger.

I read many articles about the pros and cons of the vegan diet. According to Christian Nordqvist, the vegan diet is healthy, because it reduces the risk of developing cancer, diabetes, and heart disease, as it relies heavily on whole grains, vegetables, fruits, and legumes. The difference between *pesco-vegan* diet and *pesco-vegetarian* is the addition of dairy and eggs for the vegetarians.

I owe my diet change to Tamra, my "Zen tennis friend," as I call her, for she is so composed and serene. After our tennis matches, I watched Tamra eat balanced meals, such as fresh fruit, salad, pastas without cheese, and admired her for being totally vegan. She didn't eat any meat, cheese, or sweets that contained eggs or butter, so I chose to follow her lead and turned my life around. I began to feel more energized than ever before while enjoying my crunchy and delicious salads topped with salmon, shrimp, or tofu. Our bodies do need the recommended amounts of protein (about 40-50 grams for women and about 60 grams for men, but for a more exact number, calculate the amount of protein based on your body weight). This will help your body to function properly and recover after matches.

According to the *Physicians Committee for Responsible Medicine*, the average person in the United States eats about twice the amount of protein he needs. The Recommended Dietary Allowance, or RDA, for most sedentary adults is 0.8 grams of protein per kilogram of weight. Multiply your weight in pounds by 0.36 to determine an estimate of your daily recommended protein intake. The PCRM states that "this estimate is higher than most people need, but some people, such as highly active people or women who are pregnant or breastfeeding may need more. Ask your doctor for an exact recommendation."

In one vegan food blog entitled *Health Benefits of Giving up Dairy*, the author talks about gaining weight due to her eating a lot of cheese. Once she gave up the dairy replacing it with almond milk and ate more salads, sweet potatoes, tempeh, tofu, lentils, beans, quinoa, and a variety of veggies, she lost a lot of weight and felt tremendous energy whether she went for a run, rode her bike, or taught her yoga class. The increased energy that followed her diet change made her understand why so my athletes go vegan. I can totally relate to her experience, as my endurance level is high and I feel great playing tennis tournaments for five or six hours in a row.

As Bethenny Frankel pointed out "your diet is a bank account. Good food choices are good investments." I would add that good nutrition and exercise are like a good doubles team, complimenting and supporting each other. Another reason to make nutrition an important piece of the big puzzle of good health and exercise is the discipline that a good diet brings. In another article entitled *Eat like a Buddhist in 10 Easy Steps*, Kerry Monaghan Bajaj emphasized the discipline and tenacity to adopt a vegetarian diet comprised of lentils, soups, salads, beans, etc. Other important steps were:

- follow a daily schedule for meals, no snacking.
- save dessert for a special occasion.
- enjoy home cooked meals.
- eat in silence without the distraction of television, newspaper, or radio.
- have a simple grain breakfast, such as porridge, oatmeal, or my very favorite gluten-free Muesli.

Due to the fact that these options are high fiber breakfasts and they might disagree with your stomach before matches unless you are used to eating them, I would recommend eating a high-carb breakfast, such as pancakes/waffles with jelly, or just a slice of whole grain bread with jelly. You may want to add the famous banana, which will give you potassium and might prevent you from cramping.

When it comes to cramping, Kathleen Deegan, PhD, MS, RDN, Professor of Nutrition at The University of San Francisco, pointed out some new research that classifies cramps into two distinct categories. The most common type of cramp is the EAMC, (*Exercise Associated Muscle Cramps*) caused by dehydration and electrolyte concentration. Deegan said that the famous pickle juice, contrary to a belief held by many athletes, does not alleviate cramps. However, for those tennis players who swear by it, it does not hurt to keep using it, as long as you understand that muscle cramps are caused by neuromuscular fatigue and the only cure is rest. It is also possible that nerves are wearing out from repetitive contractions, which lead to cramping.

The second type of cramp is a total body cramping, which very few people ever experience. With this type of cramp, a sodium depletion and exhaustion affects the whole body, especially people who sweat profusely, also called salty sweaters.

Another way to be prepared for your tennis matches is to balance your diet and to understand that what works for me or someone else, may not work for you. Seventy-five percent of your plate should be high quality carbohydrates, the rest should be lean meats, such as chicken, wild fish, and beans. If you are vegan, use lentils, beans, and quinoa to meet your protein needs. Yet, the guidelines that emphasize consuming less protein right before a match and having more carbohydrates, such as whole-wheat or brown rice pastas, breads, legumes, fruit (all type of berries, oranges, bananas, pineapple, watermelon, etc.) and colored vegetables, such as red bell peppers, broccoli, spinach, kale, eggplant, carrots, corn, peas, green beans, etc. are recommended.

When it comes to carbohydrates, be aware that refined carbs, such as bagels, white bread, and potatoes create a surge in insulin that in turn promotes storage of fat and may drive down your metabolic rate, says Louis Aronne, M.D., an obesity specialist at New York Presbyterian Weill Cornell Medical Center, who recommends high-fiber carbs instead. "It's important to keep carbohydrates in your overall diet, but focus on vegetables, fruits, and whole grains, which have less of an impact on insulin levels," he explains.

Another important thing you need to remember is that there are four types of carbohydrates, which is why you need to choose
wisely:

1. **Starchy carbohydrates**, such as brown rice, whole wheat pasta, sweet potatoes, old-fashioned oatmeal, corn, peas, whole wheat bread, quinoa, provide quick energy to your body and should be eaten early in the day.

2. **Non-starchy carbohydrates**, such as broccoli, Brussels sprouts, mixed greens (kale, spinach, arugula romaine), green beans, almonds, cauliflower, beets, and other vegetables besides corn and peas, are high in fiber and are best for late afternoon and early evening meals or snacks.

3. **Simple carbohydrates**, such as sports drinks and applesauce are easy to digest and are best consumed before a match.

4. **Complex carbohydrates**, such as beans that also contain fiber and protein will be harder to digest.

Knowing the difference between the types of carbohydrates you eat will make a huge difference in your body, so eat wisely and in moderation, because when it comes to calories burned vs. the ones consumed there are some important things to remember.

Let's say you run 15 miles a week and still put on weight, then think about tennis! During a regular two-set doubles match, we only run about 2 miles, so that means the caloric intake needs to be low. For instance, Christine Luff, the author of *5 Running Mistakes that Could Lead to Weight Gain* points out that 3,500 calories equals one pound, so if you need to lose the weight, you need to carefully look at the calories that your bodies need vs. calories not needed, or how to create a caloric deficit based on how many calories we burn. Luff explains that "if you're running 15 miles a week that means you're burning about 1500 calories a week (assuming you're not doing any other exercise). To get to a 3500 calorie deficit, you would need to cut 2000 calories a week, or about 280 calories per day, to lose a pound a week." And while it is not easy to figure out all our calories needs, even though USDA recommends a 2,000 daily caloric intake. Using a daily caloric expenditure calculator http://www.caloriecount.com/tools/calories-burned can give you an idea of how many calories you need on active vs. non-active days, which is also imperative to maintaining a healthy weight.

Now that you know what to eat before matches, Deegan points out that eating 30-45 minutes after a match is called the anabolic window, when the body's ability to reverse the oxidative stress and rebuild muscles is heightened. She also states that the ideal food intake after a tennis match is a 3:1 carb-to-protein ratio that will replace water and glycogen lost during the match. Deegan recommends chocolate milk as one of the best recovery drinks, because it offers a good combination of protein and carbohydrates that your body needs. The added sugar in chocolate is also essential for the muscles, as they are like sponges after exercise and will absorb and utilize those nutrients efficiently. Other foods that Deegan recommends are: string cheese, ice cream topped with fruit, yogurt-based smoothie, tart cherry juice. Sports drinks, such as Gatorade, apple slices or banana with peanut butter, and a protein bar that has 30 grams of total carbs and 10 grams of protein, are also effective for muscle recovery. Post work-outs will also help repair your muscles and reduce soreness.

A study published in the *European Journal of Nutrition* found that consuming a 100 gram bar of 70 percent dark chocolate pre-exercise reduced markers of oxidative stress post-exercise. Remember that eating a small bar or two small pieces of dark chocolate before your tennis matches will help you play better, give you more energy, and help you recover faster after long tennis matches.

Another amazing food that is a "must have" every day for tennis players and all athletes is the mighty avocado. It's packed with heart-healthy monounsaturated fats. The nutritional advantage about the avocado is that it supplies more than twenty essential nutrients, such as potassium (it has six times more potassium than a banana), copper, zinc, choline, vitamins E and K, and B vitamins. Research shows that people who make avocados part of their daily routine have a smaller waist size and lower body mass index. So go ahead and spread some avocado on your sandwiches instead of mayo or butter.

We are what we eat, so we need to become smarter about what to eat, when we eat it, and, of course, how much we eat, depending on how much we exercise. This chapter should be a constant reminder that to be great tennis players, we need to treat our bodies well and nourish them for the big matches, but most importantly for our overall health and longevity. Tennis is life and we can play it until 100!

Key points:

1. Learn as much as possible about nutrition and **eat the right foods before, during, and after matches**.

2. **Eat good quality carbohydrates**, such as brown rice pasta with marinara sauce, baked potatoes, salads, fruits, and vegetables.

3. **Stay away from greasy and fatty foods before a match**, such as a hot dog or burger. They slow down your digestion and make you sluggish, robbing you of the necessary energy needed on the court.

4. **Be smart about recovery 30 to 45 minutes after matches** and fuel your body with a 3:1 carb-to-protein ratio.

5. During matches **snack every 45 minutes, or so** to prevent your energy from going low.

6. **Sports drinks** provide the right amount of carbohydrates, sugar, and potassium to help you play longer and prevent you from cramping.

7. **Learn to make your carbohydrates your best friends**. Do not over eat bread and pastas.

8. **Learn which carbohydrates are best for you** and when to eat them. Starchy carbohydrates are better during the day and the non-starchy ones are better for dinner.

9. **Be smart about your nutrition** and enjoy longevity on and off the tennis court.

CHAPTER SEVENTEEN

Carmen's Fresh, Easy, and Healthy Menus and Recipes

"Food is our common ground, a universal experience."

James Beard

Eating healthy will translate into a faster, more energetic, and lighter you on the tennis court, which is why I have included some sample menus and recipes.

Once in a singles tournament, one of my opponents said she was feeling really sluggish and that her breakfast didn't agree with her. I was happy to share some ideas on "dos and don'ts" for breakfast I had learned. This experience made me more aware of how many tennis players struggle with nutrition. Hopefully, you will find these two chapters on nutrition and recipes helpful and easy to implement.

Breakfast sample menus:

Carmen's favorite breakfast is Gluten free Muesli (I do not have any gluten issues and do eat gluten, but I like this option for breakfast) that happens to be Djokovic's main breakfast. According to an article published in the *Tennis Magazine*, Djokovic had to make changes in his diet due to his celiac disease. A gluten free diet was one adjustment. I like to eat my Muesli with warm almond milk topped with one large tablespoon of organic peanut butter (about 7 grams of protein), fresh berries, cinnamon, and Chia seeds. I do not know how Djokovic eats his gluten free Muesli, but when I read that article, I joked with my husband and told him that I would start eating the breakfast of a champion. I was hoping his skills would rub off on me and I would play simply amazing tennis.

Top 10 healthy breakfast choices:

1. If fiber does not agree with you before matches, eat a pancake topped with jelly for quick energy and a banana. Pancakes have a little more protein than waffles, but waffles are also good choices.

2. One slice of whole grain bread topped with peanut butter and jelly and one banana.

3. If you wish to avoid any protein before the match, try whole grain bread topped with honey.

4. Scrambled eggs with bell peppers, onions, and the meat of your choice, if you need to have meat.

5. Non-sugary cereals with milk and bananas.

6. Scrambled tofu with butternut squash and spinach (recipe below).

7. A burrito with scrambled eggs.

8. Whole wheat crackers with cheese paired with a bowl of fresh strawberries, blueberries, and one banana.

9. Greek yogurt or almond yogurt topped with granola, a sprinkle of cinnamon, and fresh berries.

10. A small 10 gram protein bar (I like the kind bars with the nuts and fruit) that contains 10 grams of sugar, or less and a banana.

Additionally, I recommend eating a banana before all your matches to get the necessary potassium and to prevent muscle cramps. I also love eating two squares of dark Belgium chocolate with 72% cocoa from Trader Joe's right before a match, as research shows that dark chocolate improves your athletic performance and contains six times more antioxidants than strawberries. Another enhancer for me is the mighty green tea, which I put in my water before I play. The antioxidants in green tea are quite beneficial, so I just add two bags of tea to my cold water and I am good to go.

One year in my 4.0 league, I played a three-hour long singles match and felt so fresh in the third set, which I won 6-1.

The players from the opposite team joked with me and asked me:"What substance do you have in your water?"

"A very potent drug: green tea," I replied, and we all laughed.

After finishing your morning match, whether playing in a league or tournament, it is critical to refuel 30 minutes right after the match for fast muscle recovery.

Top 10 healthy and nourishing lunch options/menus:

1. Lentil soup, or any kind of other soup with a slice of whole grain bread, or corn tortillas. A small green salad topped with avocado, tomatoes, and nuts.

2. Turkey sandwich with green salad.

3. A bean burrito with brown rice and guacamole.

4. A peanut/almond butter and jelly sandwich, carrots, celery, and a bowl of berries.

5. Brown rice, grilled chicken, and grilled veggies.

6. Brown rice or whole-wheat spaghetti topped with marinara sauce, zucchini, red bell peppers, and fresh cilantro/parsley/basil.

7. Quick on the go lunch: chips with hummus, red bell peppers, and carrots. A 20 gram protein bar.

8. Carmen's favorite lunch after a match: Quinoa salad- (see recipe below). Quinoa is a complete source of protein.

9. A baked potato topped with marinara sauce, baked chicken, and green beans, or peas.

10. Baked sweet potatoes with wild cod and steamed broccoli.

Top 10 healthy dinners options/menus:

1. Carmen's favorite dinner: wild or brown rice with grilled/baked salmon and mixed vegetables, because of the Omega-3 fats that salmon delivers. Omega-3s can really speed up muscle recovery by reducing inflammation and potentially increasing the joint health.

2. Brown rice spaghetti with marinara sauce and zucchini.

3. Mixed greens salad topped with tomatoes, cucumbers, bell peppers, calamari olives, shrimp, sunflower seeds, olive oil and balsamic vinaigrette served with a slice of whole grain bread.

4. Miso soup and sushi.

5. Baked potato with roasted chicken or wild cod and baked fresh asparagus.

6. Chicken Chow-Mein.

7. Scrambled tofu with butternut squash and kale – (see recipe below).

8. Brown rice and roasted turkey with sautéed kale.

9. Chicken enchiladas.

10. Brown rice topped with seafood stew or Paella.

My favorite dish before or after a tennis match is: QUINOA SALAD

To prepare it, make sure you wash 2 cups of quinoa just like you wash the rice, and boil it with a teaspoon of salt for about 25 minutes till it is ready. When done, the quinoa will be fluffy just like rice. Mix the quinoa with chopped up tomatoes (two to four depending on the size), 1 red bell pepper, cilantro, 1 can of black or pinto beans, and 1 avocado. You can also add sweet corn kernels if you wish.

After mixing up these ingredients, add the juice from 1 squeezed lemon, a drizzle of olive oil, 2 tablespoons of mild or medium salsa, and voila! Your quinoa salad is ready to enjoy!

Scrambled tofu with butternut squash and kale recipe:

Cut up the butternut squash in small cubes and boil with a dash of salt. Peel the butternut squash and sautéed it in olive oil together with tofu and kale. Add turmeric, garlic, salt, and pepper at the end.

Carmen's family eggplant spread recipe - A big hit after tennis matches and at all parties:

Grill or bake 3 medium eggplants until they are very soft. Let the eggplants cool off in a bowl, after which you peel them off and cut the stem off. Leave the eggplants drain in the bowl and then drain all the bitter juices in the sink.

Use a mixer to mix the eggplants with olive oil (about two tablespoons), finely chopped onion, 1 clove of garlic, a teaspoon of sea salt, and 1 to 2 tablespoons of mayonnaise (I use the vegan type). Enjoy with pita bread or any kind of bread. It is also delicious as a side salad topped with slices of tomatoes and olives.

Brown rice pasta with zucchini and mushrooms:

Boil the pasta with a teaspoon of salt. Drain the pasta, but don't rinse it. Add cooked or uncooked zucchini, cooked mushrooms of your choice, and organic tomato basil sauce. Take it off from the stove and top it with fresh basil or cilantro.

Avocado Popsicles:

Blend together 2 avocados, 1 can of coconut milk, and juice of 1 grapefruit. Add honey to taste. Pour into popsicle molds and freeze.

Carmen's Avocado Smoothie

Blend 1 large frozen banana, 1/2 avocado, frozen berries, 1 cup of almond milk, 1 tablespoon of peanut or almond butter, a few ice cubes, a dash of cinnamon, and a handful of spinach or kale. Sip with a straw and enjoy!

Key points:

1. **You are what you eat**. Pay attention to the foods that make you feel sluggish and the ones that give you energy and stamina.

2. **Make sure to refuel 15 to 30 minutes** after matches for fast and maximum muscle recovery.

3. **Create your eating routine**. Know what foods to eat before and after a match.

4. Try different recipes. **Create a menu that is healthy, nourishing, with less animal protein and more whole grains**, such as quinoa, barley, whole wheat, as well as more fruits and vegetables.

5. **Never skimp on breakfast**. Have two or three favorite breakfast meals that will energize you and keep you full.

CHAPTER EIGHTEEN

Tips and Lessons to Take Your Tennis Game to the Next Level

"The human brain is programmed to resist change and that makes it difficult to improve your tennis game."

Online tennis instructor Florian Meyer

The moment you realize that you want to elevate your tennis game and become better at it, you should start working with a coach who can guide and teach you various shots and strategies. In my case, I had to undo a lot of bad habits. I took invaluable lessons from various tennis pros and was able to implement different shots and strategies from each coach. The ideal situation is to find a coach that will suit your greatest needs.

The goal of this chapter is to share tips from tennis coaches on what it takes to become a more proficient tennis player. I have asked each coach these questions, so each answer will match them in the exact order.

1. What is the most important thing for an aspiring tennis player to do in order to move up from one level to another?

2. What are your tips in selecting the best coach to help one's game?

3. Is there a fast track to get to higher level tennis, and if "yes", what steps should a player take?

4. What is your best tip, story, or anecdote for tennis players of all levels?

Gary Castillo, USPTA Tennis Teaching Professional at Johnson Ranch:

"First priority is to find a coach. This is needed in order to work on all your basic tennis strokes and footwork. It doesn't serve any purpose to continue practicing if you are practicing incorrectly." "Practice doesn't make perfect?" Only "perfect practice makes perfect!"

"The second priority is to find a USPTA coach that you like. It is very important to find a coach you can believe and trust in what they are teaching you. The third priority is to find a coach that makes tennis fun!"

"In order to excel quickly, you need court experience, meaning you need to play competitive matches. You can hit the tennis ball with a ball machine till you are blue in the face, but it doesn't compare to playing actual live matches. I always recommend playing against players that are a higher level than yourself. This will push your limits and make you a better player much quicker."

"This can be done by joining a Tennis Club or Public Park team and meet fellow tennis players who have the same passion as you for tennis! Surround yourself with people who love this great game of tennis! Additionally, start playing in tennis leagues and USTA sanctioned tournaments. I personally grew the most in my tennis ability by playing tournaments. There is nothing better than competing against other players to see what you are really made of inside. Many of life's lessons are discovered on the tennis court. I guarantee you will learn firsthand what's in your heart and your personal drive!"

Betsy Kessing, my very first coach, who teaches all levels at Arden Park, had the following to share:

"Take lessons from a qualified pro and play matches. The coach should be someone you feel comfortable with and understands your game and ability, so he/she can coach you appropriately." You will experience a better game "by taking lessons consistently and practicing with better levels than yourself." "Have fun!"

Jason Johnson, tennis pro at Sutter Lawn Club, added the following:

"Players need to make sure that balance and stroke fundamentals are sound. The stronger the fundamentals, the more room for progression."

"First and foremost, the person needs to make sure that the coach can get the most out of the player and vice versa. Once you reach a plateau, be willing to try lessons with others to continue your skill and strategy progression. Sometimes a different coach will provide just the key ingredient to help you pass a mental or physical block in your advancement."

"The fast track......time, time, time. Put the time in working on the fundamentals which means a lot of repetition and live ball action where you focus on execution of the basics of balance, technique, and strategy."

"My best tip would be to always be trying to become better than you were yesterday. This is a lifelong goal that with tennis can be disappointing at times when your expectations don't match with your reality. Frustration and even anger will sometimes occur when there is a dysfunction with this principal. So, set healthy goals in regards to this, and even though your journey may not be smooth, it will be a lot more enjoyable."

Martin Kosan, tennis pro at Arden Hills, where they have one of the best junior tennis programs in Northern California and where our son had the honor to train for about a year, had the following to share:

"Nothing can replace passion and hard work."

"Good personality dynamics and chemistry between a player and his coach is critical. Your coach will become a significant part of your life."

"No fast track in tennis. You try to take fast track in anything in life the results will be usually only superficial and short lasting. However, the learning curve is very individual."

"Tip: IT IS NEVER LATE TO PICK UP OR IMPROVE YOUR GAME."

Carmen's lessons learned from various tennis pros:

1. Create space between you and the ball; **do not let the ball jam you**.

2. **Use your legs to drive the ball**. Power comes from the ground. Don't be all arms trying to muscle the ball over the net.

3. **Always work on your form**, since it's hard to see ourselves have your pro videotape your moves on the court.

4. **Always check your form** whether hitting a groundstroke, a volley, or serve. Using the proper form and technique will not only improve your tennis game dramatically, but it will also reduce your risk of injuries, and who doesn't want to play tennis till 100?

5. Turn into a tree, metaphorically speaking, **plant your feet and stay grounded after running to the ball** and getting there as you hit the shot. This will translate in more consistency and more power on your shots.

6. **No lunging, no leaning!** Instead, move your feet to the ball, so that you can be in a good position to hit an effective and strong shot.

7. **Play within your means**, or your abilities, instead of trying to do something that's beyond your ability.

8. **Play and learn how to hit topspin and backspin, or slice** so that you keep the ball in and give different looks to your opponents who will have to adjust their footing.

9. **Play relaxed and find your rhythm** so that you can play long rallies when needed.

10. **Relax the wrist and release the arm** so that you can put spin on the ball.

11. **Extend your arm to finish** and follow through your shot.

12. Just like in life, **tennis is about early and proper preparation** to avoid poor performance. Turn your body early and quickly to hit the ball well.

13. **Hit your topspins from the outside leg**, which for right-handed players is the right leg, after which rotate your body and hips, or your torso to create spin and power.

14. **When hitting backhand topspin let the ball come close to you**, as reaching for it will result in losing power, or even missing your shot. When hitting slice backhands, hit through the ball without opening the face of the racket too much, as that will make your slice sit up, instead of skidding through the court.

15. **When serving, bend your knees and tilt the body** to create a heavy spin serve. Just bending the knees was huge for me as soon as I applied it to my serving motion. Don't open your body too soon; instead, stay more sideways to have a more powerful serve.

16. **When returning serve with topspin**, stay farther from the service line. Drop the racket low in a compact motion that is not as wide and loopy as the groundstroke topspin.

17. **Having a strong core is crucial in tennis**, so do your push-ups and planks every morning.

18. **Under-react, instead of over-react** any time you think you are in trouble on the court and off the court!

19. **To hit an effective and deep topspin two-handed backhand lob**, turn your body, drop the racket below the knees, and extend the left wrist for extra spin.

20. **To hit an effective topspin forehand lob**, hit the ball in front and follow through over the left shoulder.

21. **Keep your eyes fixed on the point of contact with the ball**, but don't look too early. Keep your head still, too!

22. **To execute good volleys**, turn your shoulders and hips; especially on the backhand side.

23. After hitting a wide ball, make sure to **shuffle back to the middle of the court** and anticipate your opponent's next shot.

24. Since 95% of your opponents have a weaker side, **hit to their weaker side**.

25. **Patience, spin, and placement are huge weapons** to use against heavy hitters.

Carmen's singles and doubles strategies learned from various pros:

1. **Study your opponent during practice** if playing tournaments or during the first game and make immediate mental notes and design your plan of attack.

2. When receiving a wide ball from your opponent, **hit the ball wide back.**

3. When receiving a ball in the middle of the court, **hit a high loopy topspin to your opponent's backhand and then move in to the net** quietly for an easy put away volley or overhead.

4. If your opponent has a huge forehand and runs around the backhand, **open up the court** by hitting a heavy spin ball to their forehand, after which you go down the line to their backhand.

5. **Move your opponents left and right**, and then surprise them with a shot behind them, such as hitting to their forehand, backhand, forehand, backhand, and then finishing on their backhand.

6. If your opponent is hitting every shot back, but cannot hurt you, be patient and don't try to overpower. Instead, **play a variety of shots, such as deep lobs, angles, and then look to come in to the net to finish the point.**

7. **Move your opponent's front and back by using good drop shots and then lobbing them** if they get to your drop shot.

8. **Every time you hit a good drop shot, move to the net**. Most often a drop shot is the only shot your opponent can hit from your drop shot, so be ready to anticipate this and take charge of the point.

9. **Don't allow your opponents to get set**. Instead, make them take their forehands on the run by hitting wide topspins to their forehands.

10. **On good wide shots and deep balls, move in to the net** to finish the point, but not too close by the service line.

11. **Attack their second serves by hitting deep balls to their backhands**, if backhands are weaker.

12. **Surprise your opponents to keep them guessing.** Let's say you're serving and you're leading 40-15. Serve a strong kick serve to their backhand and come to the net. Don't be afraid to serve and volley.

13. **Look to be aggressive by playing one small step inside the baseline.**

14. Try to take balls out of the air when your opponents hit floaters.

15. **Be like a chess player and design various strategies**, such as hitting to your opponents' forehand, then another forehand, and backhand.

16. **Hit to their backhand, then another backhand, and finish to their forehand.**

17. **A longer pattern would be backhand, forehand, backhand, and forehand.**

18. **Hit two heavy spin shots crosscourt and then go down the line if you managed to pull your opponent wide**, or hit another crosscourt to set yourself up before hitting a short ball or going down the line.

CHAPTER NINETEEN

The College Experience: a Faster, Fun, and Rewarding Way to Move up the Tennis Ladder

"In these days of modern tennis a player is as strong as his weakest stroke."

Bill Tilden

My passion for tennis and desire to become a more accomplished tennis player at 40 encouraged me to go back to the community college to take classes just to join the tennis team. I was driven and dedicated to change my game. I already had my Master's degree in English. When I attended college, my tennis was more for fun and recreation. Even though it would have been a great part of my curriculum, I never pursued it as a course elective.

In Fall 2013, I joined American River College regular tennis class twice a week to prepare me for the 2014 spring team tennis. I loved every hour spent on the tennis court with Reed Stout, a calm, diligent, supportive, and outstanding coach. My

18 to 20-year-old classmates were a little perplexed of this 40-year-old team mate, a mother, a professional, and an enthusiastic believer in working hard and having fun playing tennis. I enjoyed sharing court time and learning new strategies with them. I particularly enjoyed the youthful energy on the court, which made me want to run faster and hustle more to get to balls.

To be on the college team, I had to take units for the first year in tennis instruction, which was not difficult to do, since my spring tennis class counted as three units and all the rest of my classes were online. In order to be on the college team for the second year or season, you need to almost double your units, which is one of the reasons I chose to play on the team for only one season. The other reason I chose not to play a second season was my children. They had changed schools and had more extra-curricular activities. If your situation allows you to combine education with tennis that's ideal, for you can improve your tennis game while earning your degree.

Being on the college team required time, effort, and the competitive spirit to win for the team, while constantly improving and elevating my game. I practiced with the team three days a week, Monday, Wednesday, and Thursday for two hours, working on drills, serving, playing matches, doing conditioning, talking strategy, and planning for our matches.

Tuesday and Friday were our match days when we played one singles and one doubles match against local college teams, such as Sierra College, Folsom College, as well as Santa Rosa, San Francisco, to name just a few. Home matches were my favorite, as I lived 10 minutes away from American River College and biked to school. Our away matches took all day, but I was fortunate to have my husband help me with our children, picking them up from school, feeding them, and putting them to bed, as I usually got home around 9 p.m. When we had away matches we received a small lunch and dinner allowance from the athletic department. After a long day of tennis and traveling, we had dinner together and talked about our matches, our experiences, what went well and not so well. We laughed a lot, even when we had a tough loss on the courts.

I was surrounded by young, energetic, and exuberant team mates who loved tennis, which gave me more energy and drive to improve my game. On my end, I took the time to encourage and inspire my younger team mates. At the end of our season, I received an award for being the most inspirational player for phenomenal participation on the American River College Women's Tennis - 2014 season. My life experience, my energetic personality, and my competitive spirit all helped the team. I knew we could all aspire for more, work harder, train smarter, eat healthier (I used to make a delicious Quinoa salad that I would bring and share with the girls and our coach), and be more confident on and off the courts.

We only had seven players on the team that season, so I got to play all the matches. I finished with a record of 9 wins, 6 losses. I had a few singles matches that I won 6-0, 6-0, because my opponents did not know how to handle my slice. I lost matches from players with big topspins and a consistent game. The team finished second in the *Big 8 North Conference* and fifth in Northern California.

Playing tennis on a community college team is definitely an attainable goal for players of all ages, especially for women, as most of the college teams do not have enough players. The men teams are more impacted and harder to get into. The difference between the women's teams and men's teams is the NTRP level. For instance, in the women's teams there are players ranging from 3.00 to 4.5, but in the men's teams they range from 4.00 to 5.00, so it is more competitive.

10 steps to get into a community college and play on the tennis team:

1. **Contact the tennis team coach of the college** (info is on the college website under the athletic department) you wish to attend based on proximity to your home, the tennis program they have, or your educational goals.

2. If you know someone on the tennis team, **have that person introduce you to the coach.**

3. **If you played NTRP tournaments and USTA league matches**, tell the coach. Many college players do not have a lot of match experience and this experience will make you a great addition to the team.

4. **Being athletic helps** to train every day, but I have heard of women in their 60s who played on the college team and did really well, so if you are ready to get to the next level and love tennis, by all means join the tennis team and also broaden your education or knowledge by taking classes.

5. **Sign up for classes and take online classes** that are easy for you if you are not pursuing a degree. For a degree, you will need to take regular and online classes, but it you are doing

this from the tennis perspective, then have fun and pick classes that you will enjoy.

6. **First semester take the tennis class twice a week** to get a feel of how things work.

7. **Work diligently, be flexible** and be ready to learn new things.

8. Second semester is tennis season, so team training happens every day and you will have two matches a week, most weeks. Training is not hard, but having good stamina helps, so **eat healthy, sleep well, and bring your energy on the court.**

9. During tennis season, or the spring semester, which starts in January till May (tennis training and competition ends by April) with matches starting in February, there are **two important tournaments against other colleges**, which are a lot of fun and provide great competition, so be ready to be away from home for two days or three depending on the tournament and location.

10. **Be ready to cross train**, such as light running, lifting weights, doing stretches and yoga, which will all improve your tennis game and reduce your risk of injuries!

After getting accepted on the college team, it is up to you as a person and player to make the college experience great. I immediately realized that being old enough to be my team mates' mother, I still needed to blend in. First, I observed the dynamics around me. Then, I absorbed things and became more flexible and open-minded to the way I approached my game and interacted with my team mates.

The most valuable advice I can give you is to be ready to change your game, since that's the big reason you are there. While working hard on your game, help your team mates do the same by being supportive and inspiring. Stay positive at all times and do not let losses dampen your spirit. Instead, learn from your mistakes and losses and do your best. The wins will follow for sure, especially if you become aware what went well and not so well in your matches. A good way to remember is to keep notes about your tennis progress, as well as jot down tennis tips and strategies from your coach.

After the work is completed, remember to eat and sleep well before every match, as well as hydrate well before, during, and after matches. And last, but not least: **HAVE FUN!**

CHAPTER TWENTY

The PR of Tennis

"If you can't fly then run, if you can't run then walk, if you can't walk then crawl, but whatever you do you have to keep moving forward."

Martin Luther King, Jr.

After I provided you with a comprehensive tennis guide, compendium, or just your tennis bible, I figured you would want to know how to PR in tennis, which stands for personal record. As opposed to running, when I strive to run faster and beat my slower time from a previous race, a PR in tennis stands for **perseverance, patience, practice, and results**.

Perseverance is that indomitable spirit that if we keep striking the fuzzy yellow ball, we will become better players. It is also a trait that trickles over to our lives when we properly connect the dots between hard work and proficiency. Our tennis shots feel easier to execute and our whole beings get to marvel at the first key word forming the PR of tennis. In my case, learning topspin forehand took a lot of perseverance, as I had to keep hitting balls that felt more alien to me than my coming to America and leaving my old country Romania behind. With tennis, I was simply leaving my slices to lurk between the familiar and unfamiliar. I treaded over unchartered territories and cringed at my inconsistency when executing my new shots. Yet, better be uncomfortable than remain a dinosaur. It is better to fail in the beginning, while prevailing at the end, which pretty much sums up what it takes to persevere.

Patience requires time and dedication. To me, patience simply means brushing up on our tennis strokes the same way my father dusted off the hands of time when repairing watches. He was a watchmaker and he could sit hours cleaning, dusting, and repairing the old mechanisms of his customers' watches. He was also the most patient man I have ever met, as he never complained about how long it took him to do something. On the contrary, he thought repairing a watch in four hours was not too long and that he needed to take his time to fix the time of his customers – pun intended.

I was fortunate to work side by side with my dear father when I was in middle school. I learned to brush the watches, which is why brushing up the ball in tennis reminds me about my father's old watches that needed so much cleaning and care. Taking time to brush up our tennis skills simply requires patience and time, as things definitely do not happen overnight. Thus, when you hear your coach tell you that learning a new stroke, or changing something in your game takes time, remember patience as a quintessential component of the tennis PR, and you will PR for sure in due time.

Practice, our third "p" in our PR chase is strongly intertwined with perseverance and patience. When we strive to learn something new, we need to practice so much more than when executing shots that we are already comfortable and familiar with. In tennis, practice can be quite difficult, especially when a player plays a lot of competitive matches. That's the reason we need to set aside time to practice with a good partner who also wants to try new strokes, strategies, and just play differently than in competitive matches when we are less likely to employ and deploy new shots. Moreover, playing against a player who is a little weaker, or at a lower tennis level than yourself can be quite beneficial, as it makes it easier to practice new shots. Conversely, playing against a player who is higher ranked than yourself is also ideal, for it totally forces you out of your comfort level and pushes you to try things, since you have nothing to lose. In 2015 when I used to play so many competitive league and tournament matches and got moved up to the 4.5 level, making time to practice was difficult, but I still managed to do it once a week, which gave me more confidence to try my topspin or my sliced backhands during matches.

Results make our tennis PR sweet and intoxicating. The "r" stands for results, which feels like reaching the top of the mountain at the end of a long, arduous hike. Unlike running, when results are evident by seconds and minutes, in tennis, results can take years. Thus, being patient will make our tennis PR sweeter and more enjoyable, even though it would be more gratifying to have faster results with less work and dedication, but then life would be too easy and even boring.

Just like in running, tennis PRs can happen one after another, especially when we break down goals and make them realistic. One way to celebrate our tennis PRs is to keep notes on the results we want to see after taking lessons for a month, three months, etc. Writing down specific goals, such as "I want to develop a more effective backhand slice that will stay low and will be hard to attack," or "I want to use more topspin lobs after I bring my opponents to the net," will equate a tennis PR, which should be celebrated.

Key Points:

1. **Running around the tennis court with a goal in mind** and not just chasing the fuzzy yellow ball can result in a PR.

2. **When you persevere**, you make time your friend and become a more accomplished tennis player and human being.

3. **Practice with a purpose** and the rewards will be forthcoming.

4. **Results can vary depending on your PR expectations.** They can be more evident in the beginning when you keep improving, but they can also stall for a while until you do something else to your game.

5. **Think about the PR both on and off the tennis court**, as perseverance, patience, and practice will lead to other successful practices in your life, earning you many medals like the ones I earned in over 20 running races.

6. **Results are concrete measurements of your hard work**, but do not solely rely on whether you win or lose a match. Instead, analyze what you did better than previous matches.

7. **Losing in tennis means that you can still PR** based on how you performed in the match, since a 5-7, 6-7 loss means that you performed well and you still achieved a PR.

8. **Learn to analyze your losses and your wins** to determine your next PR.

9. **Enjoy the journey and be patient**! It all comes together sooner or later.

10. **Celebrate the journey to your PRs** rather than just the PRs; it's more rewarding.

CHAPTER TWENTY-ONE

Carmen's 100 Life Lessons

"Fall over seven times, and get up eight."

Japanese proverb

In the past 20 years, I have played over 100 tennis tournaments ranging from 3.5 level to open. I have played singles, women's doubles and mixed doubles, and have always learned something new about tennis, people, and life, which is why I have decided to create my own special list of life's lessons learned through tennis.

1. Be fair, and then check your fairness once again.

2. Breathe, inhale, and exhale.

3. Don't ever give up on yourself and your dreams!

4. Chase anything that resembles a yellow fuzzy ball. The fuzzier the better, as it will allow for exploration.

5. Don't ever pout, but some grunting is allowed, especially when tired to release the trapped energy.

6. Don't lunge for something that does not belong to you. You'll miss, or hit the net.

7. Don't reach and grab, unless you are reaching for someone's hand.

8. Wait patiently for the right moment.

9. Measure your steps.

10. Jump rope.

11. Run between 2 to 10 miles a couple of times a week for a stronger body and mind.

12. Practice yoga for a flexible body and mind.

13. Hike in nature alone and with friends.

14. Stop to smell the flowers.

15. Write poems and haikus.

16. Keep a diary.

17. Take notes to remember things later, as well as to spark up new ideas.

18. Read and read some more.

19. Learn something new every day.

20. Associate yourself with the doers, not the naysayers.

21. Have meaningful and stimulating conversations.

22. Keep small talk to a minimum.

23. Look at the bigger picture.

24. Study.

25. Work hard.

26. Train hard.

27. Under-promise and over-deliver.

28. Be honest.

29. Don't lie unless you have to save a friend's life.

30. Recover.

31. Retrain your mind.

32. Retrain your eyes to really see.

33. Change to become the best YOU!

34. Don't expect others to change for you.

35. Accept people the way they are.

36. Do not judge!

37. Do not gossip!

38. Do not point fingers, or blame!

39. Take responsibility for your own actions.

40. Admit your mistakes.

41. Become smarter about your mistakes.

42. Learn from your mistakes.

43. Don't repeat your mistakes.

44. Do things differently!

45. Embrace your perfectly flawed SELF!

46. Continue on the road less traveled.

47. Stay on the path.

48. Put one foot in front of the other.

49. Fall 100 times (I fell 100 times before I learned how to ski), and then get up again.

50. Don't look back!

51. Always look forward!

52. Look over your shoulder for just a second, and then know where to go and how to position yourself in a favorable situation.

53. Don't linger.

54. Be ready to split step and volley life's problems with a strong core and set of beliefs.

55. Smile, shake hand, and compliment the other person.

56. Put other people's needs first.

57. Make people smile.

58. Make people laugh.

59. Do not be a bore!

60. Be interesting!

61. Be curious!

62. Be observant!

63. Be ready to change and adapt to the situation.

64. Ask questions.

65. Give genuine praises.

66. Encourage others to reach their highest potential.

67. Be inspirational to others!

68. Be supportive!
69. Have confidence in yourself.
70. Instill confidence in others.
71. Live with a "can do" attitude!
72. Know that everything is possible when you have faith in yourself!
73. Live a full life!
74. Treasure life's beautiful moments!
75. Travel to new places as often as you can.
76. "Step into the ball," means take charge in life when you need to.
77. "Go around the ball," means don't let life's problems jam and crush your spirit.
78. "Early preparation," means just that: get prepared early to be well-positioned in life.
79. Since tennis requires a geometric thinking, this means look at life from all angles and relish your discoveries.
80. Use different lenses to grasp life's hidden gems.
81. Do not criticize!
82. Do not nitpick!
83. Be a good listener.
84. Talk less, and listen more.
85. Hug more!
86. Be kind!

87. Be warm and generous!

88. Be humble!

89. Stay grounded!

90. Keep your cool!

91. Develop a constant "joie de vivre," or, in other words, enjoy life.

92. Just like in tennis, be a good server in life by helping others.

93. Celebrate your Aces in tennis and your As in life!

94. Look to contribute to a bigger cause.

95. Do not brag! Let your results speak for you!

96. Do not envy someone who is better or has more than you; instead work hard to be like that person!

97. Always be open to constructive criticism, as it is the only way you can grow!

98. Be open to try new things!

99. Be yourself, as everyone else is already taken!

100. Stop competing against others! Choose instead to compete against yourself to become the best YOU!

CHAPTER TWENTY-TWO

Tennis Resources

"Champions keep playing until they get it right."

Billie Jean King

Tennis resources for Northern California, United States, and International players Colleges - applying for their tennis programs

With change comes disruption, which is why I ask you to ponder on the following question: "How can we disrupt our complacency and satisfaction with things we do on all levels of our lives?" One way is by gently pushing ourselves to do more and to require more of ourselves, as we are all perfectly capable of reaching higher professional, fitness, intellectual, and any other goals we set our minds on achieving. Another way is by being balanced. To me, balance is the constant intertwining of time and space, of work and pleasure, of family and friends, of new and old, of learning and changing, of growing and helping others change their grip on life.

Speaking of growth and change, I have had the honor and privilege to interview Kent Kinnear, Director, Player ID and Development with the United States Tennis Association National. Here are the questions I had for Kinnear regarding the junior development programs and their grants opportunities:

"What can you tell us about your Junior development program?"

"USTA (United States Tennis Association) National works closely with each section to provide a training pathway that includes orange and green ball camps for players 7-10 years old (Early Development Camps, or EDCs), as well as Team USA Sectional, Regional, and National camps for players 11-14. These are for the top players from the section. From there, a smaller number of players from around the country can qualify to be on the TEAM USA Summer National Teams, which also include possible training opportunities with USTA National Coaches at our National Training Centers," Kinnear stated.

"How can parents apply for tennis scholarships and programs for their children?

"The camps mentioned above are not designed to be applied for – the players are selected based on feedback and information shared from each section's Coaches Commission, which is a group of coaches who are located around the section, attending tournaments, and providing feedback on players they have observed. We encourage the commission members to not go just by rankings and ratings, but also take into consideration if the player might be a multi-sport athlete, possibly under-resourced, or very new to the game. The exception to this are the multi-cultural grants available through the Diversity and Inclusion Department. These are grants that need to be applied for. The criteria for those multicultural grants are available online."

"What are the criteria for a junior tennis player to be considered for a scholarship or grant through the USTA Junior Development Program?"

Kinnear said that USTA Sections have certain grant money that they distribute, whereas the multicultural grants are given by the Diversity and Inclusion Department. He added that at national level, there are no scholarships offered, but there are different types of grants that they offer to offset tournament or coaching expenses. Moreover, these are only available for the players at the highest level of each birth year from 13 and older. There are two main type of grants explained below:

1. **Excellence Grants** awarded to junior and professional players 20 years old and younger eligible to receive up to $9,000 per year through USTA Player Development's Excellence Grants, which are awarded solely on merit, via rankings or results. For complete information and necessary forms visit: www.usta.com/playergrants.

2. **Grand Slam Grants** awarded to players who are accepted into and compete in the singles main draw of the Australian Open Jrs., French Open Jrs., and Wimbledon Jr. Championships. These players will receive a travel grant: $1,750 for the Australian Open; $1,250 for the French Open and Wimbledon. Grants will also be awarded to players who qualify for the main draw in singles of any of the above listed

Junior Grand Slams. No grant is given for the U.S. Open Junior Championships.

And last, but not least, I asked Kinnear about **USTA's future plans regarding promoting the junior tennis and having more opportunities for talented juniors.**

"We will continue to work with the private sector coaches and sections as part of the TEAM USA collaboration and provide a training pathway of EDC camps and TEAM USA Camps and Teams to help increase the opportunities to a wide base of young players. We will also provide additional opportunities for training, trips, and national teams for players in their teenage years that begin to be more based on results at tournaments nationally and internationally."

With all the opportunities that tennis has to offer on a physical, mental, emotional, and spiritual level, my question to you is: "Got grip?" If you do, adjust it, change it, and tweak it to get a better grip on life and tennis, while venturing outside of your homes, your worlds, and your comfort zone. Remember to open your hearts and souls to new possibilities and continue to explore life with curiosity, joy, excitement, mindfulness, balance, and awareness.

I hope you have enjoyed reading the book and that you can apply some of the advice to take your game to the next level.

Please purchase this book for yourself and all your tennis and non-tennis friends who value sports, exercise, good nutrition, and a new grip on life.

With every book sold, USTA (United States Tennis Association) receives $1 to go towards the development of their junior tennis scholarships and programs.

Special Offers

FOR A COMPREHENSIVE 1-HOUR SMALL FEE: TENNIS CONSULTATION WITH ME REGARDING YOUR TENNIS, FITNESS, AND LIFE GOALS. FEEL FREE TO CONTACT ME AT CARMENMICSA@YAHOO.COM, OR CALL ME AT 916-342-2446.

BONUS 1: Purchase four books or more, and receive the fifth one at half the price. For tennis lessons on implementing some of the ideas in this book, please contact the following tennis coaches mentioned below, and receive $10 off your first 1-hour lesson.

BONUS 2: Purchase 10 books, or more, and receive a special pricing discount.

Betsy Kessing, Tennis Pro at Arden Park
Jason Johnson, Tennis Pro Sutter Lawn Club
Gary Castillo, USPTA Tennis Teaching Professional at Johnson Ranch
Amine Khalid, USPTA Tennis Teaching Professional at Gold River Racket Club
Milun Doskovic Doskovic, USPTA Tennis Professional at Gold River Racket Club
Glen Davis, USPTA Tennis Teaching Professional at Natomas Racket Club
Reed Stout, former coach of the women team at American River College
Martin Kosan, Tennis coach at Arden Hills

Joe Gilbert, Head Pro of Arden Hills Junior Tennis Academy

Other valuable resources for tennis players:

United States Tennis Association, our most valuable resource: the association that sets up all our league divisions, tournaments for juniors and adults, and so much more.

https://www.usta.com/
http://www.norcal.usta.com/adultleagues/

Courtside Tennis, the place to get all your tennis equipment, apparel, shoes, etc. with three locations in Gold River, Sacramento, and Roseville.

http://www.courtsidetennis.com/

For those players looking to be stylish and very comfortable when playing tennis, check out **B-Passionit** clothes designed by two local tennis players and amazing business women, Denise Antoniades and Lisa Podlipnik. You can find their clothes at Courtside Tennis, as well as on their website.

www.bpassionit.com.

American River College, where you can join the tennis program and team and train hard to get to the next level.

http://www.arc.losrios.edu/

Symmetry for Health if you need help alleviating those back pains, or any other pains.

www.symmetryforhealth.com

Works Cited

http://www.mindbodygreen.com/0-6425/Eat-Like-a-Buddhist-in-10-Easy-Steps.html, Bajaj, Kerry Monaghan, *Eat like a Buddhist in 10 Easy Steps*, Oct. 10, 2012

http://www.yogajournal.com/slideshow/yoga-athletes-4-poses-tennis/#slide-0, Cruikshank, Tiffany, *Yoga for Athletes: Four Poses for Tennis Players*, Aug. 3, 2015

http://news.yahoo.com/10-foods-fight-inflammation-090000502.html, Largeman-Roth, Frances, *10 Foods that Fight Inflammation*, March 23, 2015

Levey, Jon, "The Grip Guide," *Tennis*, March/April 2016

http://running.about.com/od/strengthtraining/fl/Strengthening-Workouts-for-Runners.htm, Luff, Christine, *Strengthening Workouts for Runners*, July 31, 2015

http://running.about.com/od/RunningandWeightLossTips/ss/Running-Mistakes-That-Could-Lead-to-Weight-Gain.htm#step2, Luff, Christine, *5 Running Mistakes that Could Lead to Weight Gain*, July 31, 2015

http://www.active.com/tennis/Articles/8-Lunges-to-Improve-Tennis-Fitness.htm, McGee Suzanna, *8 Lunges to Improve Tennis Fitness*, March 25, 2015

http://www.mindbodygreen.com/0-17072/the-only-4-moves-you-need-for-a-strong-core.html, Powell, Chris, *The Only 4 Moves You Need for a Strong Core*, Jan. 23, 2015 http://www.livestrong.com/article/556190-protein-content-in-mushrooms-vs-meat/, Sarka-Jonae Miller, Feb. 24, 2015

http://www.popsugar.com/fitness/Health-Benefits-Giving-Up-Dairy-35694882, Sugar, Jenny, *6 THINGS that Happened When I gave up Dairy*, 2/21/2015

http://play.babolat.us/increase-tennis-serve-speed-video?email=carmenmicsa@yahoo.com&utm_source=hs_email&utm_medium=email&utm_content=24922850&_hsenc=p2ANqtz-_WpgkbtxdW32tEewAg8b5LM1pmTOTAxz8-g96OpK_4mSlaVP2myedi7FCC3yM8arajKDSUq8G2sfWkY76ZmwkiV5Crlg&_hsmi=24922850, Salzenstein, Jeff, *Increase Your Serve Speed*

https://www.yahoo.com/health/5-habits-of-vegetarians-you-should-steal-114423947803.html?soc_src=unv-sh&soc_trk=fb&fb_ref=Default, Sas, Cynthia, *5 Habits of Vegetarians You Should Steal*, March 31, 2015

http://www.mindbodygreen.com/0-13415/5-reasons-to-do-burpees-every-day.html, Stryker, Krista, *5 Reasons to do Burpees Every Day*, April 20, 2014

http://www.active.com/page34314.aspx?PageMode=Print, Van Der Meer, Dennis, *7 Steps to a Perfect Serve*, April 28, 2012

http://www.medicalnewstoday.com/articles/149636.php, Nordqvist, Christian, *Vegan Diet: Health Benefits of Being Vegan*, Dec. 2, 2015

About the Author

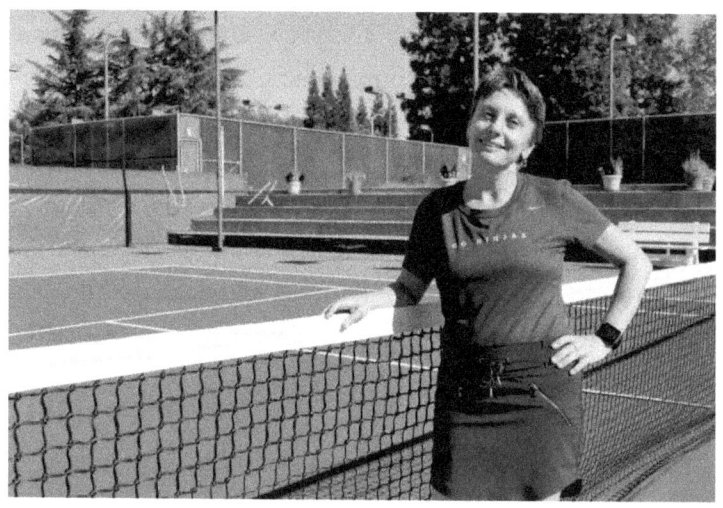

Born and raised in Romania, Carmen Micsa moved to America in 1995 and chose to write about her old life in communist Romania and her new life in America. *Freedom Rocks* is Carmen's first book/memoir that she is also working on publishing. She has published articles in a few local and national publications and a memoir piece *Grandpa's Garden* in the anthology *From Sac Home Myths & Other Untruths* together with some of her graduate school classmates. Carmen also writes short fiction, travel articles, and picture books. She is also the owner/author of her blog www.runningforreal estate.com.

She earned a BA degree in English and a MA in English (Creative Writing) both from Sacramento State University.

Besides writing, Carmen Micsa enjoys being a mother to her two beautiful children Alex and Sophia. She owns her own real estate company, Dynamic Real Estate and prides herself for being organized and efficient in leading a balanced life.

Carmen continues to excel as a competitor. She finished number two in Northern California in women singles as a 4.00 in 2015 and got moved up to 4.5. She also ran her third marathon in 2016, the California International Marathon in Sacramento, which she finished in 3:47:47 minutes with a personal best. Besides tennis, Carmen loves to bike and has done 100K and century (100 miles) bike rides for Diabetes Tour de Cure in memory of her beloved father. Her enthusiasm and energy branch into her various life roles as a dedicated mother, wife, daughter, writer, real estate broker, tennis player, runner, and friend.

Carmen can be reached via her website www.carmenmicsabooks.com. You can also email her at carmenmicsa@yahoo.com. Her Facebook page is www.facebook.com/cmicsa.